...tents

Acknowledgements

We are grateful to many people for their advice and assistance, particularly to Dr Elisabeth Whipp, FRCR, Consultant Clinical Oncologist at the Bristol Oncology Centre; Dr J. Boyle, FRCP, Consultant Dermatologist, Musgrove Park Hosptial, Taunton, Somerset; Kate Westbrook, Radiography Services Manager, Bristol Oncology Centre; Dr Tim Mitchell, GP; and Ward Sister Stephanie Saunders, Frenchay Hospital, Bristol. Thanks are also due to Louise Smith, Radiographer at the Bristol Oncology Centre, to Marlene Mackay, and to the men and women who told us of their experiences for the section of case histories.

General preface to the series

Two people having the same operation can have quite different experiences, but one feeling that is common to many is that things might have been easier if they had had a better idea of what to expect. Some people are reluctant to ask questions, and many forget what they are told, sometimes because they are anxious, and sometimes because they do not really understand the explanations they are given.

The emphasis in most medical centres in Britain today is more on patient involvement than at any time in the past. It is now generally accepted that it is important for people to understand what their treatment entails, both in terms of reducing their stress and thus aiding their recovery, and of making their care more straightforward for the medical staff involved.

The books in this series have been written with the aim of giving people comprehensive information about each of the medical conditions covered, about the treatment they are likely to be offered, and about what may happen during their post-operative recovery period. Armed with this knowledge, you should have the confidence to question, and to take part in the decisions made.

Going in to hospital for the first time can be a daunting experience, and therefore the books describe the procedures involved, and identify and explain the roles of the hospital staff with whom you are likely to come into contact.

Anaesthesia is explained in general terms, and the options

available for a particular operation are described in each book.

There may be complications following any operation – usually minor but none the less worrying for the person involved – and the common ones are described and explained. Now that less time is spent in hospital following most non-emergency oper-ations, knowing what to expect in the days following surgery, and what to do if a complication does arise, is more important than ever before.

Where relevant, the books include a section of exercises and advice to help you to get back to normal and to deal with the everyday activities which can be difficult or painful in the first few days after an operation.

Doctors and nurses, like members of any profession, use a jar-gon, and they often forget that many of the terms that are famil-iar to them are not part of everyday language for most of us. Care has been taken to make the books easily understandable by everyone, and each book has a list of simple explanations of the medical terms you may come across.

Most doctors and nurses are more than willing to explain and to discuss problems with patients, but they often assume that if you do not ask questions, you either do not want to know or you know already. Questions and answers are given in every book to help you to draw up your own list to take with you when you see your family doctor or consultant.

Each book also has a section of case histories of people who have actually experienced the particular operation themselves. These are included to give you an idea of the problems which can arise, problems which may sometimes seem relatively trivial to others but which can be distressing to those directly concerned.

Although the majority of people are satisfied with the medical care they receive, things can go wrong. If you do feel you need to make a complaint about something that happened, or did not happen, during your treatment, each book has a section which deals in detail with how to go about this.

It was the intention in writing these books to help to take some of the worry out of having an operation. It is not knowing what to expect, and the feeling of being involved in some process over which we have no control, and which we do not fully understand, that makes us anxious. The books in the series *Your Operation* should help to remove some of that anxiety and make you feel less like a car being serviced, and more like part of the team of people who are working together to cure your medical problem and put you back on the road to health.

You may not know *all* there is to know about a particular condition when you have read the book related to it, but you will know more than enough to prepare yourself for your operation. You may decide you do not want to go ahead with surgery. Although this is not the authors' intention, they will be happy that you have been given enough information to feel confident to make your own decision, and to take an active part in your own care. After all, it is *your* operation.

Jane Smith
Bristol, 1996

Preface

Most skin cancers are caused by excessive exposure to ultra-violet radiation from the sun and are therefore preventable. Some occur in later life as a result of sun damage to the skin during childhood. Tanning of the skin is the visible evidence of damage to it and is caused by the increased production of pigment as the skin tries to protect itself. Although the risk is greater in countries near the Equator and in the Southern Hemisphere, prolonged exposure to the sun in more temperate climates, even on cloudy days, can cause sunburn and skin cancers. Sun-related skin cancers are most common in those with fair or freckled skin and far less common in black races.

Although this book explains the treatments and operations for skin cancers once they have developed, it is hoped that the information it contains will also raise people's awareness of how to reduce their risk of developing these diseases and of how to detect the signs of skin cancers already present. Early detection and treatment improve the prognosis for almost all types of skin cancer and can play a significant role in reducing mortality rates for the most serious form – malignant melanoma.

Over the last few decades, we have come to equate a suntan with good health, but this is a view which has to be revised if we are to reverse the current trend of an increasing incidence of skin cancers in many countries. We can help to reduce the future incidence if we take sensible precautions to protect ourselves and, perhaps more importantly, our children and to educate them about the risks involved.

Jane Smith
John Kenealy
Bristol, 1996

CHAPTER 1

Introduction

WHAT IS A CANCER?

A cancer is a group of malignant cells which are not subject to the normal controlling mechanisms of growth, reproduction and death and which, if left untreated, will eventually spread locally and possibly also to other parts of the body. The cancer at the original site is called a **primary** and that which develops following spread of the cancer cells is a **secondary**.

Although the word **tumour** is often used to mean a cancer, a tumour is strictly a swelling, which can be either malignant or benign, whereas skin cancers can be flat or even ulcerated and are therefore more accurately described as **malignant skin lesions**. A skin lesion is any area of abnormal skin, whether benign or malignant, which is the result of damage or injury or which has changed its function or appearance. We have therefore used the term lesion rather than tumour throughout this book, except in a few instances when specifically referring to a swelling.

Spread of cancer cells occurs via the blood or lymphatic vessels. The lymphatic vessels transport **lymph**, a pale-coloured fluid which contains disease-fighting cells called **lymphocytes**. At various sites throughout the body there are glands called **lymph nodes** into which the lymph drains. The lymph nodes in the immediate vicinity of a skin cancer – the **regional nodes** – are often involved in the early stages of cancer spread. The process of spread of malignant cells is known as **metastasis**, and the secondary cancers which develop as **metastases**.

Not all skin cancers metastasise, and those which do not are usually relatively simple to treat, particularly if detected early. But when metastasis of a skin cancer does occur, the malignant lesions which develop in other body organs can be the cause of more serious illness. Very occasionally a skin cancer shows spontaneous remission, for reasons which are not yet understood.

Unlike malignant lesions, benign lesions do not spread, but remain localised at the site at which they develop. They are not life threatening, are unlikely to recur once they have been completely excised, and are usually quite simple to treat. There are several different benign skin lesions (see p.4), as well as some which have the potential to become malignant (see p.6).

The book deals primarily with the three main types of skin cancer: **basal cell carcinoma**, **squamous cell carcinoma** and **malignant melanoma**. But first it may be helpful to have some knowledge of the structure and function of the skin itself and of the variety of benign skin lesions which can occur.

THE HUMAN SKIN

The skin forms an almost continuous outer covering to the body, acting as a container and helping to protect the internal organs from mechanical injury and invasion by bacteria. It also regulates the body's temperature and helps prevent it dehydrating. It consists of a thinner outer **epidermis** and a thicker inner **dermis** which is attached to the underlying body structures by strands of connective tissue. Underneath the dermis is a layer of subcutaneous fat which varies in thickness throughout the body.

The epidermis

The epidermis does not contain blood vessels, and its living cells receive nutrients from fluid which leaks from the blood vessels within the dermis. Its thickness varies on different parts of

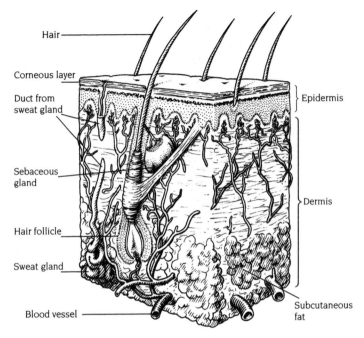

Hair

Corneous layer

Duct from
sweat gland

Sebaceous
gland

Hair follicle

Sweat gland

Blood vessel

Epidermis

Dermis

Subcutaneous
fat

The human skin.

the body: it is thickest on the soles of the feet and on the palms
of the hands.

The epidermis has a basement layer of **basal cells** which
become flattened **squamous cells** as they migrate upwards
towards the surface of the skin. The innermost layer of the epidermis is the **malpighian layer** which contains cells called
melanocytes. The melanocytes produce granules of pigment,
called **melanin**, which give the skin its colour. The melanin is
taken up by **keratinocytes** within the dermis, and these cells
divide and migrate upwards through the epidermis to form an
outer, tougher, horny layer of dead cells which are continuously
rubbed off and replaced from below.

The dermis

The fibrous tissue of the dermis contains nerve endings, blood and lymphatic vessels, organs which sense touch, pain and changes in temperature, sweat and sebaceous glands, and hair follicles. Ducts from the sweat glands pass through the epidermis and open in tiny pores on the surface of the skin. The sweat glands secrete water containing small amounts of salt and other waste products, which evaporates from the surface of the skin and helps regulate the body temperature. The sebaceous glands secrete an oily substance called sebum which lubricates and protects the hair and skin surface and reduces the evaporation of water from the cells, preventing dehydration.

BENIGN SKIN LESIONS

There are many benign skin lesions, and although most are quite easily identified, some can resemble malignant skin lesions and may need to be differentiated from them. Brief details are given below of the most common. (The names in parentheses are alternatives which you may come across.) Other, less common, types include adenomas (lesions of the sebaceous and sweat glands), atypical fibroxanthomas (lesions composed of fat-rich cells), granulomas (lesions of granulation tissue) and cysts (fluid-filled cavities).

* Naevi (*pigmented moles*). There are many different types of benign naevi, varying in size, shape and colour, some of which contain hairs. The following are the three main categories.
* *Junctional naevi* often develop in children before puberty as dark brown or black, flat lesions anywhere on the body. They may eventually transform into compound or intradermal naevi (see below), and there are claims that they can become malignant.

4

* *Compound naevi* are most common after puberty and are usually small, brown or black, nodular lesions surrounded by a brown ring. They may be hairy. Although compound naevi can become malignant, they are more likely to evolve into the intradermal type.
* *Intradermal naevi* are the most common moles in adults. They often develop on the scalp or face as flat or nodular, pigmented or colourless, often hairy lesions of any size. They very rarely become malignant.

Although benign lesions often alter with time, *any change in an existing mole*, especially in its shape or colour, ulceration, bleeding, itching or inflammation may be an indication of malignancy which should be reported to your doctor. *Any new mole* which is different in appearance from existing ones should also be seen by your doctor. If there is any doubt, the mole can be excised and examined under a microscope for the presence of cancer cells.

* *Basal cell papillomas (seborrhoeic keratoses, senile warts, seborrhoeic warts)*. These are raised, wart-like lesions which vary in colour from pale to black. They occur most commonly on the face, shoulders, chest or back of middle-aged or elderly people. Although benign, they can be unsightly and are sometimes removed for cosmetic reasons.
* *Haemangiomas*. These vascular lesions can develop in a variety of forms. They may occasionally give rise to concern if they are small and dark in colour, resembling a malignant melanoma to the naked eye. However, when viewed under magnification, the two are easily distinguished.
* *Solar lentigos (senile lentigos)*. These are very large freckles which develop as brown patches on the skin in response to damage by the sun. Lentigos are flat and often occur on the backs of the hands or wrists in elderly people.
* *Keloids*. These are swellings of fibrous scar tissue which often

develop at the site of a scar or injury and are usually easy to identify. They seem to be more common in black races and can be disfiguring.

* *Dermatofibromas* (*sclerosing angiomas*). These small, usually pink-coloured, dome-shaped growths often develop at the site of an insect bite, particularly on the arms or legs. Darker-coloured dermatofibromas may resemble malignant melanomas, especially when surrounded by a pigmented ring.

* *Keratoacanthomas*. Although most common on the face, these lesions can also occur on the arms and hands. They grow quite quickly but always resolve spontaneously after a few months, sometimes leaving a scar. They can be difficult to distinguish from squamous cell carcinomas and therefore always need to be investigated. A lesion diagnosed as a keratoacanthoma but which persists for longer than a few months without showing signs of spontaneous healing is probably a squamous cell carcinoma.

LESIONS WITH MALIGNANT POTENTIAL

There are some apparently benign skin lesions which will need to be monitored as they can transform into cancer. Examples include *giant congenital naevi* (present from birth) and *dysplastic naevi*. The latter are atypical, distinctive lesions, the presence of which increases an individual's risk of developing malignant melanoma by more than tenfold.

More common are the *actinic keratoses* (*solar keratoses, sun warts*). These rough-textured lesions can be pink or brown, and occasionally transform into squamous cell carcinomas (see p.10), although they rarely metastasise. On becoming malignant, they will enlarge, bleed or ulcerate. Actinic keratoses are most common in fair-skinned people and develop in skin which is exposed to the sun, for example on the face, neck, hands, arms and legs.

SKIN CANCERS

Most skin cancers are caused by excessive exposure of the skin to the sun, with or without prior sensitisation by chemicals or other agents. There are two main categories of skin cancer: carcinomas and melanomas.

A **carcinoma** is a cancer in epithelial tissue, such as the skin and the lining of most of the body's hollow organs. Carcinomas are always malignant, but they can vary in severity. The two most common types of carcinoma of the skin (which will be dealt with in this book) are the basal and squamous cell carcinomas. Superficial skin carcinomas such as **intra-dermal carcinomas** can be treated by a variety of methods such as scraping, freezing or simple excision (see p.34). Intra-epidermal carcinomas are slowly expanding, pink, scaly malignant lesions which develop as non-invasive forms of basal or squamous cell carcinomas, the latter known as **Bowen's disease**. More deep-rooted lesions may require surgery or radiotherapy. Treatment at an early stage is successful in 95 per cent of cases. Although together these two types of carcinoma account for about 10 per cent of all types of cancer, they are the cause of only 0.3 per cent of cancer deaths.

The third, more serious, type of skin cancer is malignant melanoma. A **melanoma** is a cancer of melanocytes (see p.3) which is usually, but not always, pigmented. Malignant melanoma will eventually metastasise, either locally or to distant sites, if left untreated.

Less common skin cancers

Apart from the three most common types of skin cancer mentioned above, and dealt with in detail in this book, there are several other forms which are less common. Briefly, they include the following.

Lymphomas are cancers arising in lymphoid tissue, and include Hodgkin's disease and a condition known as mycosis fungoides. Skin cancers may develop as primary or secondary manifestations of a lymphoma.

Sarcomas are relatively rare cancers of connective tissue. **Kaposi's sarcoma** is a bleeding cancer which occurs particularly on the lower legs and feet. One type is most common in elderly men of Mediterranean or Jewish descent, another is endemic in central, equatorial Africa, and another can arise following immunosuppression therapy for organ transplantation. These cancers often develop slowly, but there are more aggressive forms which can involve the internal organs, for example one which is associated with AIDS and HIV infection and which now occurs in endemic areas.

Basal cell carcinoma

Basal cell carcinomas (also known as **rodent ulcers** because of their rather gnawed-looking centre) are the most common type of skin cancer, accounting for about 80 per cent of all cases. They develop in the lower basal layer of the epidermis and are slow-growing, relatively superficial lesions which are sometimes present for many years before medical advice is sought. If left untreated, they can penetrate deeper into the skin, eventually causing damage to underlying cartilage and bone.

Basal cell carcinomas tend to arise on areas of the skin exposed to the sun, particularly those with a high concentration of sebaceous glands, such as on and around the nose, temple and forehead. Although they do not normally recur after apparent complete surgical excision or radiotherapy, they can do so. Basal cell carcinomas on the side of the nose immediately adjacent to the eye or at the base of the nose where it joins the cheek tend to be particularly prone to recurrence, which may be because they are aggressive forms or may result from the fact that their location means that only a limited margin of surrounding normal skin can be excised or irradiated.

Basal cell carcinomas *per se* very rarely metastasise, but a variant form with features of both a basal and a squamous cell carcinoma (commonly known as a **basi-squamous**) has a much higher rate of metastatic spread and of local recurrence, tending to be clinically more aggressive than either of the derivative forms.

There are several different types of basal cell carcinoma which can usually be distinguished by an experienced specialist.

* *Nodular (papulonodular)*. This is the most common type of basal cell carcinoma, a well-circumscribed, pearly lesion with overlying fine blood vessels which may bleed during the later stages of development. It may be raised above the skin and, as it grows, may develop a small central area of ulceration. Nodular basal cell carcinomas may be microscopically solid or cystic.
* *Cicatricial (sclerosing)*. This type of basal cell carcinoma has a more diffuse margin, and often spreads across the skin without obvious thickening. It may have a central scarred appearance, with active growth only at the periphery, and may become quite extensive, eventually covering several centimetres or more.
* *Pigmented*. This type of basal cell carcinoma has features similar to the nodular type, but a more irregular outline and pattern of pigmentation. The lesions can sometimes be confused with malignant melanomas, although the distribution of the pigment within the two types is different, and clinical differentiation is usually possible.
* *Morphoeic*. These basal cell carcinomas become apparent as ill-defined, whitish changes in the skin and spread superficially. They are a rarer form of the disease and occur almost exclusively on the face.

* *Infiltrating.* Infiltrating basal cell carcinomas can occur in various forms, as red, grey or whitish lesions which may ulcerate. On microscopic examination, they may be found to have infiltrated to some depth.
* *Multi-focal.* A multi-focal basal cell carcinoma may develop as a red patch of skin with a pearly margin, possibly with a central white area. It may be superficial or have invaded to some depth by the time medical attention is sought.

Treatment

Thin basal cell carcinomas can often be frozen (by **cryosurgery** or **cryotherapy**, see p.37); thicker ones will probably have to be scraped out (by **curettage**, see p.36) or cut out (by **surgical excision**, see p.36). Sometimes radiotherapy is used for someone who is elderly or unfit and for whom surgery is inadvisable.

Following the excision of a large cancer, a skin graft or flap repair may be necessary. Very large basal cell carcinomas sometimes require more complex reconstructive procedures. The various operations are explained in Chapter 6.

The prognosis following treatment of basal cell carcinomas is generally good, but they very occasionally prove fatal if they remain untreated or are particularly aggressive. Aggressive forms in the head or neck region may eventually invade vital areas such as the cranium, causing more serious problems.

Squamous cell carcinoma

About 15 per cent of skin cancers are squamous cell carcinomas. They can arise anywhere on the body where there is an epithelial surface. Those on the skin mainly occur in sun-exposed areas, such as the face and hands, but they can develop on the legs, particularly in women who tend to expose their legs to the sun more than men. However, skin cancers on the leg are often basal cell carcinomas.

Although relatively slow growing, squamous cell carcinomas develop more rapidly than basal cell carcinomas and occasionally metastasise. If left untreated, they will eventually penetrate deeper into the skin, and often arise in areas with definite signs of sun damage and solar keratosis (see p.6). They almost always ulcerate at an early stage but may be covered with wart-like scaly skin. Their growth may be predominantly upwards or they may ulcerate into the skin.

Treatment

In the very early stages of development, before they have become invasive, squamous cell carcinomas can be treated by topical agents such as 5-fluorouracil, by cryosurgery or cryotherapy (see p.37), or by excision and direct closure of the skin. Once invasion has occurred, they are generally best treated by surgical excision, although radiotherapy may be appropriate when surgery is inadvisable. As squamous cell carcinomas are usually more invasive and have more diffuse margins than basal cell carcinomas, a wider surrounding area of tissue is normally excised, and therefore reconstruction with skin grafts or flaps is often required (see Chapter 6).

Like basal cell carcinomas, squamous cell carcinomas generally have an excellent prognosis following treatment.

Malignant melanoma

Although often referred to simply as melanomas, all melanomas are malignant, i.e. a type of skin cancer. They account for about 5 per cent of all skin cancers and are most common in people of Celtic origin, and in those with red hair, fair skin and freckles. Like most types of skin cancer, they are rare in black races. The tendency to develop this type of cancer may be genetic – it sometimes occurs in several members of the same family – although environmental factors probably play the most important role.

Occasionally a melanoma is only detected following discovery of a secondary cancer in a regional lymph node, and there may sometimes be more than one melanoma present on the body. Careful examination of someone with a melanoma or cancer of the lymph nodes is therefore necessary to preclude these possibilities.

There are four main types of malignant melanoma, as well as a few rare varieties.

* *Superficial spreading*. This is the most common type of melanoma (constituting about 75 per cent of all types). It often occurs on the legs of women and the bodies of men in their forties and fifties. Superficial spreading melanomas tend to have an indistinct edge and irregular pigmentation, possibly with blue, black or pink patches. Initially flat, they may become raised when advanced.
* *Nodular*. Nodular melanomas appear to develop more quickly than the superficial spreading type and become raised at an early stage of development. They account for about 15 per cent of all melanomas. They are most common in late middle age, occurring on the body, head, neck or, in women, the legs. Unlike other melanomas, they are often uniform in colour, being blue, grey or black, although they can be almost colourless. Their outline is more regular and their surface is smooth, although an ulcer may develop at an early stage which may be accompanied by bleeding.
* *Lentigo maligna*. This is arguably the least malignant type of melanoma. It often develops on the faces of elderly people or on other parts of the body regularly exposed to the sun. Lentigo maligna melanomas make up about 7 per cent of all melanomas. They are initially flat, have an irregular brownish pigmentation and grow slowly, over several years. They have an irregular outline and may show thickening and the development of nodules at a late stage.

* *Acral lentiginous.* This is the least common type (about 3 per cent), except in Japan and in African races whose incidence is approximately equal to that of other races but for whom this is probably the most common type of melanoma. The lesions develop on the palms of the hands and soles of the feet, particularly in dark-skinned people, and sometimes under the nails. Although they may be large, it is often some time before medical advice is sought as they may be mistaken for a blister or wart. This type of melanoma often develops as a brownish black lesion which eventually becomes raised and ulcerated.

Development and spread

There are two main stages in the development of a malignant melanoma. During the first, the cancer remains **in situ**, tending to grow horizontally. A melanoma diagnosed and treated at this stage has an extremely good prognosis and very rarely metastasises. The next stage of melanoma development is the **invasive** stage, during which the cancer starts to grow downwards into the skin. Once it becomes invasive, it tends to grow progressively deeper, and the prognosis becomes progressively worse.

In general, melanomas are symptomless until a relatively late stage. Itching, bleeding and ulceration tend to occur late in their development, if at all. They seldom cause pain or discomfort.

When metastasis of a melanoma occurs, it usually does so first via the lymphatic system (see p.1), the malignant cells spreading to the local regional lymph nodes. Later on, and also occasionally as a first step with some melanomas, spread occurs via the blood to any site in the body, most commonly the liver, brain and lungs and sometimes the bones.

Assessing the prognosis

There are two commonly used methods of assessing the prognosis of a malignant melanoma based on microscopic examination of its tissue. **Clark's method** involves assessing the level of invasion of the cancer in relation to the skin structures. The developmental stages are numbered from 1 to 5, level 1 being in situ and level 5 being the most invasive stage. **Breslow's method** correlates better with prognosis and is based on measurement of the thickness of the cancer in millimetres from the granular basal layer of the epidermis. The melanomas are categorised as thin, intermediate or thick, with corresponding deterioration in prognosis. A melanoma with a large surface area does not necessarily give more cause for concern than a smaller one. It is the *depth of invasion* rather than the horizontal spread of the cancer that has most affect on the outcome.

Prognosis is also affected by whether or not the melanoma has ulcerated, its rate of growth, its site, and the sex and general health of the individual, as well as by whether or not it has spread at the time of diagnosis. The outcome is generally better for women than it is for men, and a melanoma on the leg has a better prognosis than one on the trunk, head or neck. Therefore, all other things being equal, a woman with a melanoma on her leg tends to have the best prognosis.

Treatment

The treatment options are dealt with in detail in the appropriate chapters. But briefly it can be said that, provided it is feasible, surgery is usually the treatment of choice for both primary and secondary malignant melanomas. Various additional treatments have been (and are still being) tried in combination with surgery, including chemotherapy, immune therapy and radio-therapy for secondary cancers. However, none has yet been shown to improve long-term survival, although many are of palliative value in the short term, relieving symptoms when cure is not possible.

Surgery of a primary melanoma involves excising the malignant tissue together with a margin of surrounding normal tissue. This treatment is based on historical evidence which indicated that it resulted in relatively fewer local recurrences.

Individual surgical practices vary, but a common one is to excise a centimetre of tissue on either side of the cancer for every millimetre of its depth, up to a maximum of 3 cm. Direct closure of the wound is usually possible when a margin of up to 1 cm has been excised, but for excisions larger than this, either a graft or flap repair is required. Excision and direct closure can often be done using a local anaesthetic and as day-case surgery (see p.41). A wider excision normally involves in-patient treatment, with a post-operative stay ranging from a day for large flaps to a week or more for skin grafts, depending on the site of the cancer.

RISK FACTORS

There are various factors associated with an increased risk of developing skin cancer, but the most significant is excess exposure to ultraviolet radiation. There are also certain categories of people who are at greater risk, for example those with large numbers of acquired moles (i.e. moles which have developed since birth). It may be that these people are particularly susceptible to ultraviolet radiation and that their moles have developed as a response to it. Some 5 to 10 per cent of people who develop a malignant melanoma have a family history of the disease, but whether this is due to a shared gene or a shared environment cannot be certain. There are some familial conditions, such as familial atypical mole syndrome, which are associated with a higher incidence of malignant melanoma.

Advice about how to reduce your risk of developing skin cancer is given in Chapter 2.

Ultraviolet radiation

The cause of many skin cancers – and probably the major cause of malignant melanoma – is excessive exposure of the skin to the ultraviolet (UV) rays of the sun. Radiation from the sun is known as electromagnetic radiation, and includes radiation of

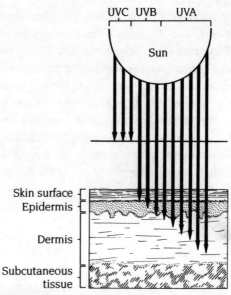

UVC UVB UVA

Sun

Skin surface
Epidermis

Dermis

Subcutaneous
tissue

Ultraviolet radiation. This diagram shows how far the different types of ultraviolet radiation penetrate into the skin.

very high frequency and therefore short wavelength and high energy, such as ultraviolet radiation. Only a very small amount of the sun's total radiation reaches the earth, as most is absorbed or scattered as it passes through the atmosphere, particularly in the ozone layer surrounding the earth.

Ultraviolet radiation is made up of rays beyond the visible spectrum of light, and although it is necessary for some processes of normal growth, excessive exposure not only ages the skin but causes permanent damage. It consists of UVA, UVB and UVC. Only the first two are present in natural sunlight, as UVC does not penetrate the ozone layer. Ultraviolet B rays are responsible for the actual burning of the skin, but there is now little doubt that UVA rays are also harmful. However, there is at present some controversy about the specific effects of the different types of ultraviolet rays.

Although it is very difficult to ascertain risk factors with any degree of certainty, it does seem likely that people with most exposure to ultraviolet light, whether constant or intermittent, are most at risk. The cumulative dose of ultraviolet radiation is certainly important in the development of basal and squamous cell carcinomas, but excessive intermittent exposure may be more relevant in malignant melanoma.

Data from Australia indicate that the higher incidence of **non-melanocytic** skin cancers (i.e. those other than malignant melanoma) in men in that country may be related to the fact that more men than women work outside. Some studies show a higher incidence of malignant melanoma in women and in indoor workers whose exposure to the sun is intermittent, often leading to sunburn.

Another Australian study indicated that people who emigrate there before the age of 15 adopt its high risk of developing malignant melanoma. Those who emigrate to Australia after the age of 15 retain the risk of their country of origin. The data suggest that it is exposure to the sun (and any other relevant risk factors) during *childhood* which is crucial in the development of this type of skin cancer.

Other factors or combinations of factors may sensitise an individual to the carcinogenic effects of ultraviolet rays. For example, infection of an immune-suppressed person with the human papilloma virus (which causes warts) may lead them to develop squamous cell carcinoma after sun exposure.

The effects of ultraviolet radiation are discussed further in Chapter 2.

Genetic disorders

There are several congenital disorders which are associated with an increased risk of developing skin cancer following sun exposure. People born with Gorlin's syndrome may develop basal cell carcinomas in their teens or twenties. Congenital sebaceous naevi can turn into basal cell carcinomas at a similar age.

Another, rare, congenital condition, xeroderma pigmentosa, involves a defect in the ability of cells to repair their DNA when it is damaged, for example by ultraviolet radiation. People with this condition are sensitive to sunlight and at high risk of developing basal and squamous cell carcinomas.

There are other congenital disorders associated with an increased risk of malignant melanoma, including familial atypical naevus syndrome and giant congenital hairy naevi.

Chronic irritants

Although now mostly of historical interest, there are various factors which can predispose to pre-malignancy and which have been the cause of skin cancer in the past. The use of aniline dyes by leather workers and the exposure of chimney sweeps to coal tar, for example, contributed towards the occurrence of scrotal skin cancer in people in these jobs.

Skin cancers of the lips can occur in heavy smokers, and are common in certain countries where the chewing of beetel nuts is prevalent.

Ulcers and trauma

Rarely, squamous cell carcinomas can arise in areas of the body with chronic ulceration, such as the legs. Even more rarely, they can develop in scar tissue which has formed as a result of trauma or burning etc.

Radiation

Skin cancer developed in some people 30 or 40 years after they had received radiotherapy to treat ringworm, a treatment which is no longer used. Although much more stringent precautions are now taken with the use of X-rays, radiotherapy for skin cancer is really a more suitable treatment for older people as it can have harmful effects in the long term (perhaps after 20 years or more) similar to those caused by ultraviolet radiation.

Immunosuppression

Squamous cell carcinomas may develop as a result of exposure to ultraviolet radiation following suppression of the immune system by drugs, for example after kidney transplantation.

INCIDENCE OF SKIN CANCER

The reported incidence of skin cancer has increased in recent years – by over 80 per cent in the UK during the last ten years. Although all skin cancers are most common after the age of 50, malignant melanoma can occur in younger people and, rarely, in children. Skin cancer is the most common cancer in the Southern Hemisphere. Its incidence is highest in countries at low latitude which are inhabited by white people, for example Texas, USA, South Africa, Australia and New Zealand, and doubles with every ten-degree decrease in latitude. However, other factors may play a role, such as in Norway where the incidence is three times that in France and twice that in Britain, despite its higher latitude. Also, for example, the very high incidence of skin cancer in Queensland, Australia (40 in every 100 000 inhabitants), may be more directly related to its being a coastal region. It may also be partially explained by the fact that many of Queensland's residents have ancestors from Britain who migrated there in the late 1700s. In doing so, these fair-skinned Europeans moved some 20 degrees closer to the Equator and significantly increased their risk of skin cancer.

Malignant melanoma

Recent figures show that New Zealand now has the highest rate of death due to malignant melanoma in the world: 8 men and 4 women in every 100 000 of the population.

There is a low incidence of malignant melanoma in Japan and Hong Kong, where it affects about 0.2 people in every 100 000. Approximately 10 in 100 000 people develop the disease in the UK, where its incidence is increasing by about 1.7 per cent each year. As malignant melanoma is thought to be largely preventable, it may become less prevalent in the future as people become more aware of the importance of avoiding excess exposure to the sun, particularly in children.

Basal and squamous cell carcinomas

Basal and squamous cell carcinomas cause a relatively small number of deaths each year, most of which are the result of complications due to metastasis of squamous cell carcinoma or to its direct invasion of vital structures.

SKIN CANCER IN CHILDREN

Although skin cancers can occur in children under the age of 14, they rarely do so. However, sunburn during childhood seems to be linked to melanoma in later life, and children should always be protected from exposure to the sun.

Basal cell carcinomas sometimes develop in congenital lesions in children, such as in sebaceous naevi or giant cell naevi, and very rarely without any such obvious association. Squamous cell carcinomas rarely occur in teenagers who have been exposed to the sun at a very early age, but they are extremely rare in younger children.

About 0.3 per cent of malignant melanomas occur in children

under the age of 14, most in giant congenital hairy naevi. Melanomas may be more common in those with a large number of moles, although at least 50 per cent arise *de novo* (i.e. not in a pre-existing mole).

Prevention

The majority of cases of skin cancer are caused by excessive exposure to the sun, and are therefore preventable. This chapter explains how to take sensible precautions to protect your skin against the damaging effects of the sun's rays, and thus reduce your risk of developing skin cancer. Tanning of the skin is a protective mechanism – the skin's response to damage – and there is no such thing as 'safe sun exposure'. The only way to avoid the risk of sun-induced skin cancer completely is to keep your skin covered. The skin can burn in cool, cloudy conditions, it simply takes longer than in hot, sunny weather.

PEOPLE AT INCREASED RISK

The darker your natural colouring, the lower your probable risk of developing sun-related skin cancer. Although everyone should protect their skin from sunburn, it is particularly important for people at higher risk, especially children (see p.20) and those with:

* fair or freckled skin or skin which burns easily;
* red or fair hair and light-coloured eyes;
* a large number of normal moles;
* large, irregularly shaped or irregularly pigmented moles;
* a history of severe sunburn, particularly during childhood;
* a history of malignant melanoma;
* other family members who have had malignant melanoma;
* certain hereditary conditions (see p.17).

PROTECTING THE SKIN FROM SUNBURN

Until about the middle of this century, it was fashionable to have pale skin. Men and women wore clothing which covered most of their body, and almost everyone wore a wide-brimmed hat. After the Second World War, clothes became a bit more revealing and swimming costumes came into fashion. Hats were smaller, and eventually it became acceptable not to wear one at all. Foreign holidays to hot countries were more generally accessible, and seaside holidays and swimming in the sea started to become popular. At the same time, tanned skin began to be considered desirable.

Although by the 1930s skin cancer was starting to be a real cause for concern, it was not until the 1950s that the role of the sun in malignant melanoma was first appreciated.

The darker skinned indigenous people of many hot countries, whose risk of developing skin cancer is lower than that of people with fair skin, are well aware of how to avoid the dangers of the sun. They may have a siesta in the early afternoon, and will certainly try to stay indoors or in the shade in the middle of the day when the heat from the sun (and the ultraviolet radiation level) is most intense. Similar precautions are sensible for everyone, especially during the summer months.

* *Always avoid the sun during the middle of the day when it is at its strongest.* The sun is strongest between the hours of 10 in the morning and 2 in the afternoon. The intensity of ultraviolet radiation depends on the distance it has travelled through the atmosphere: the lower the angle of the sun above the horizon, the greater the distance it has to travel and the less intense it is. At noon in the summer, the sun is directly overhead and the ultraviolet radiation has its shortest passage through the atmosphere.

The greater the distance from the equator, the lower the sun reaches in the sky at midday in the winter and thus the lower the

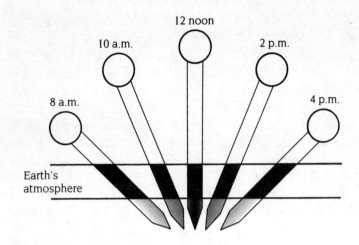

Avoid the sun around midday. A proportion of ultraviolet radiation from the sun is absorbed as it passes through the earth's atmosphere. As its path through the atmosphere is shortest between the hours of 10 a.m. and 2 p.m., the sun is strongest during this period.

level of ultraviolet radiation. However, it is possible for the skin to be burnt by the sun at any time of the year, even in temperate climates; it just takes longer when the sun is less intense. The sun is stronger at the top of a mountain than it is at sea level, and therefore it is possible to get sunburn at altitude even in winter, particularly when ultraviolet radiation is reflected off snow or water.

Thus it should be remembered that the dose of ultraviolet radiation received by the skin depends not only on the strength of that radiation, but also on the duration of exposure to it.

*   *Cover your skin when in the sun*. When you are out in the sun, you should cover your shoulders, arms and legs with loose-

fitting clothing made of tightly woven material, even in overcast, breezy conditions. Cotton protects the skin and helps to keep you cool. Always wear a hat with a wide brim to protect your face. Do not expose the same area of skin for a long period and be careful not to fall asleep in the sun without first covering yourself up.

As the sun's rays are reflected off water and sand (as well as off buildings and pavements), you can get sunburnt on a beach under a beach umbrella.

*   *Use a sunscreen preparation appropriate for your skin type.* Melanin absorbs ultraviolet radiation, and its content in the skin increases in response to sun exposure – resulting in a suntan. Apart from darkening to try to protect itself from sun damage, the skin also thickens and produces sweat to absorb ultraviolet radiation. But the body is unable to protect against intense exposure, and there are various sunscreen preparations available for those who have to be exposed to the sun. Sunscreen preparations provide useful additional protection for people who work outdoors or who take part in outside sports such as golf, tennis or watersports, but their use should not be seen as a means of enabling 'safe sunbathing'.

Some sunscreen preparations provide a block to ultraviolet radiation by covering the skin in an opaque, insoluble film (often white or coloured) which forms a physical barrier to both UVA and UVB. Sunblocks help prevent tanning and burning of the skin, but as they reduce the loss of sweat from the body, they may cause discomfort if applied all over and are therefore usually used on the nose, lips, ears etc.

The sunscreens which are more widely used absorb the energy from ultraviolet radiation before it can reach the epidermis. Unlike the sun blocks, these chemicals are not visible when on the skin surface. Use a preparation which protects against UVA and UVB.

Sunscreen preparations have sun protection factors (SPFs) which are a measure of the amount of protection they afford. In general, the higher the SPF, the longer you can stay in the sun without burning your skin. For example, if you know that the first signs of sunburn appear after 10 minutes of exposure, a sunscreen with an SPF of 10 may enable you to stay in the sun ten times as long, i.e. 100 minutes, before burning starts. Someone whose skin starts to burn after 20 minutes can use a product with an SPF of 5 to enable them to remain in the sun for the same length of time (100 minutes). If you have freckled or sensitive skin which burns easily, fair or red hair, you will need a preparation with an SPF of at least 15. If your skin tans easily without burning, a lower SPF may be adequate, although the more the skin is screened the better, whatever your skin type. However, sweat washes off some sunscreen preparations faster than others, and all creams or lotions should be applied regularly – at least every two hours and after swimming. Sensitive areas – such as the lips, eyelids, nose, cheeks, chest, shoulders, nipples and soles of your feet – should be kept well protected.

There are also various 'suntan preparations' available which contain a chemical which reacts with chemicals in the skin to produce a colour resembling a tan. They do *not* provide protection to the skin unless they have an SPF value, and only those which do provide sunscreening should be used.

Recent information from the National Radiological Protection Board suggests that the doubling of the annual rate of malignant melanoma in Britain in the last 15 years (to approximately 10 new cases per 100 000 people) may have been contributed to by the fact that people spend longer in the sun when they think they are protected by a sun cream or lotion. When used correctly, sunscreen preparations allow you to stay longer in the sun before your skin burns, but they do not give complete protection from all types of ultraviolet radiation. The constituents of sunscreen preparations made in some countries may also actually increase the risk of skin cancer.

*   *Gradually increase the time you spend in the sun.* If you really must get a suntan, you may be able to reduce the dose of ultraviolet radiation by *gradually* increasing the time your skin is exposed over a period of several days. But remember, **there is no safe dose of ultraviolet radiation**. You should never leave your skin exposed to the sun until it turns red, as by the time it does so the damage will have already been done. The most dangerous type of sun exposure, particularly for the young, is sudden, short and intense, and malignant melanoma may be linked to severe sunburn while on holiday.

*   *Protect children from the sun.* There is increasing evidence indicating that sunburn in childhood is linked to melanoma in later life. Protecting children from sunburn is therefore essential. Children's skin is very delicate and children of all ages should wear loose cotton clothing made of densely woven fabric, hats with wide brims, sunglasses, and sunscreen preparations when out in the sun. Small babies should be kept out of the sun completely. Those older than six months should only be exposed for short periods, and should always be protected by a sun preparation of at least factor 15.

*   *Protect your eyes.* Apart from causing skin cancer, the sun can also damage the eyes, so you should wear *good* sunglasses in bright sunlight. In Britain, sunglasses have to conform to a British Standard so that their lenses filter out harmful rays from the sun. If you normally wear spectacles, you should have purpose-made prescription sunglasses rather than simply tinting the lenses of your spectacles, which does not have the same protective effect and may, in fact, be damaging as they cause the pupils to dilate, thus exposing the lens of the eye to more ultraviolet light. Good sunglasses are particularly important for children.

SUNBEDS

Ultraviolet A rays are responsible for the ageing of the skin; ultraviolet B rays cause sunburn and seem to play the major role in inducing malignant changes. Until relatively recently, sunbeds were generally considered to be safer than direct exposure to the sun as they apparently use more ultraviolet A than B rays. However, evidence now suggests that this claim is controversial.

There is no such thing as safe ultraviolet radiation, and although certain bands of the ultraviolet spectrum are more damaging than others, they are all damaging to some extent. The use of sunbeds increases the cumulative dose of ultraviolet radiation, and therefore most doctors would now advise against them. Sunbeds may increase the risk of cancer and their regular use certainly damages the skin. In fact, recent evidence seems to indicate that the use of a sunbed before exposure to the sun may increase your risk of skin cancer, although the reason why this should be so is not yet apparent.

SELF-EXAMINATION

Self-examination is particularly important for people whose risk of developing skin cancer is increased for some reason (see p.22).

Detection of the early signs of skin cancer has an important part to play in controlling the disease. Regularly examining your skin will help you to be aware of any changes which could be significant (see p.5). Learn where your moles and birthmarks are, inspect them regularly, perhaps monthly, and look for new ones which are different from the existing ones.

Having removed all your clothing, use both a hand-held and a full-length mirror in a well-lit room to examine every part of your body. You may need to ask a friend or family member to help you if, for example, you are unable to see all of your back clearly.

If you are in any doubt about whether an existing skin lesion has grown or changed in some way, it is useful to be able to compare it against an earlier photograph in which it is visible.

CHAPTER 3

Investigations and treatment options

SYMPTOMS AND SIGNS

A **symptom** is a disturbance in the normal working of the body which is not necessarily visible but which is felt by the patient, for example itching. A **sign** is something a doctor looks for as evidence of disease or medical abnormality, such as bleeding or swelling.

If you have several moles or other skin lesions which look the same, the chances of them all being malignant are very low, regardless of their appearance. However, if *one* of them changes in appearance or size, there is more reason for concern.

It is important not only to be aware of any changes in existing moles or other skin lesions – such as in their size, shape or colour – but also of the development of new ones, and to seek medical advice at an early stage. Although many people know that changes in existing moles should be investigated, it is perhaps less widely known that at least 50 per cent of malignant melanomas and nearly all other skin cancers arise spontaneously as new lesions on areas of previously clear skin. Even when changes in existing lesions do occur, some 80 per cent are still benign and alter because they have become infected or have been irritated, for example by the sun or by rubbing. Although itching and bleeding are not necessarily indications of malignancy, they can be be relatively late signs that a skin lesion has become cancerous. (Melanomas are usually, but not always, brown to black in colour.)

VISITING YOUR FAMILY DOCTOR

If you visit your family doctor because you are concerned about a skin lesion, the action taken will depend in part on his or her experience of skin cancers. Experienced doctors are often able to recognise skin malignancies by their visual appearance, but some refer almost all skin lesions for a specialist opinion. The type of specialist you see will depend to some extent on who is available in your area. Diagnosis will be based on the site of the lesion, whether or not it is pigmented, its size, shape and texture, and whether it has changed suddenly in appearance or size.

You should be prepared to give your doctor a history of your skin lesion, and it may be a good idea to look at some old photographs of yourself for evidence of how long it has been present, how much it has grown, and whether or not it has changed in appearance. If possible, you should take any useful photographs with you when you go for your appointment.

Your doctor will look carefully at your skin lesion, and may measure it, making a note of any relevant details. If there is any doubt about whether it is a new growth or whether it has been present for some time but has changed in appearance, you may be referred for specialist advice. If your doctor is confident that the lesion looks benign and has not altered with time, you may be asked to return at a later date so that it can be checked again, or you may be referred to a specialist to confirm the diagnosis.

If you are very anxious, and your doctor is experienced in performing minor surgery, he or she may decide to put your mind at rest by removing the lesion, probably at another appointment and using a local anaesthetic. If the wound is closed with non-absorbable stitches, these may be removed after about seven days by the practice nurse. The surgical excision of any lesion will leave a scar, which will be longer than the lesion itself. Any excised tissue should always be sent to a laboratory for examination under a microscope.

VISITING A SPECIALIST

You may be referred by your doctor to a dermatologist, plastic surgeon or clinical oncologist (see below). In some areas, there are joint skin clinics staffed by some or all of these specialists, and the services available in your area will largely determine to which type of doctor you are referred. Some dermatologists now also practise minor reconstructive surgery, which will be necessary after the removal of a large lesion or one in certain sites of the body. Non-melanoma skin cancers may sometimes be referred directly for radiotherapy, particularly those in older people.

Doctors specialise in different areas of medicine at registrar level (see p.47), and it may be useful to have an idea of the different specialists who treat skin cancers.

* **Dermatologists** have specialised in diseases of the skin (and probably also in venereal diseases). They are mainly physicians but have varying degrees of surgical experience.
* **Surgeons** have specialised in diagnosis, disease processes and the practice of surgery. A surgeon can become a specialist in a specific type of surgery, such as plastic or vascular surgery, or in general surgery. Surgeons are the only specialists to be known as Mister or Miss when they become consultants.
* **Oncologists** are physicians who have specialist training in all aspects of cancer, particularly radiotherapy and chemotherapy, but not surgery.

The specialist to whom you are referred will examine your skin lesion and question you about its history in much the same way as your family doctor.

32

Although the tissue from any potential skin cancer must be examined under a microscope to confirm the diagnosis, it is unlikely that a surgeon will do a biopsy of a basal or squamous cell carcinoma at your first out-patient appointment. If there is any doubt about the identity of a particular lesion, it will have to be completely removed and tissue from it will be histologically examined once this has been done (see p.34).

A dermatologist, on the other hand, may do an incision biopsy (see below) of a basal cell carcinoma so that its tissue can be examined and the diagnosis confirmed, before removing it by excision, burning, scraping or freezing.

Scans and blood tests are not usually necessary for diagnosis, although they may be done if metastasis is suspected.

Most people with a skin lesion who are referred to a specialist can be reassured that it is benign and does not require any treatment. Some will be asked to return in a few months time so that their lesion can be examined again.

CLINICAL TESTS

Incision biopsy

As has been mentioned above, there are some instances in which a biopsy will be done, either before or during treatment. An incision biopsy involves cutting away a small slice of the lesion and normal tissue once the area has been numbed by the injection of a local anaesthetic. The small wound may be left open to heal or it may be closed with a couple of stitches.

Melanomas are very rarely biopsied. Although incising a melanoma does not affect the prognosis, it does prevent a complete specimen being available to the pathologist, which may lead to potential inaccuracies in the measurement of its depth of invasion (see p.13).

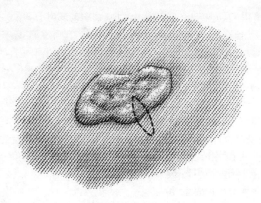

Incision biopsy. The dotted line indicates the area of malignant and normal tissue which might be removed for histological examination.

Cytological examination

Some skin lesions exude a fluid, a sample of which can be obtained by pressing a microscope slide onto the surface of the skin. The sample can then be examined under a microscope for any sign of cancer cells.

Histological examination

A histological examination involves looking at tissue, rather than at cells. The whole cancer or a small sample of tissue is removed by biopsy and sent to the laboratory to be examined under a microscope. All excised skin lesions should be examined histologically.

TREATMENT OPTIONS

The main consideration when planning treatment is to excise the skin lesion completely, but whenever possible cosmetic appearance should also be taken into account. You will be offered the treatment which is thought to be most appropriate for you, although the choice is inevitably also influenced by the particular experience of the specialists in your area. You may want to ask if you can talk to more than one type of specialist (surgeon, radiotherapist, dermatologist) if you are concerned about a particular type of treatment.

Dermatologists normally treat small skin growths, although an increasing number are now becoming experienced in the techniques of minor reconstructive surgery and some are experienced at excising larger lesions and repairing the skin with grafts or flaps. Plastic and reconstructive surgeons excise small lesions on cosmetically obvious areas and larger ones which require reconstruction of the surrounding area of skin. Radiotherapists treat cancers with radiation, which is generally more appropriate for older people and for those with lesions which cannot be reached surgically without causing damage to adjacent body parts. Radiotherapy is rarely suitable for treating malignant melanomas but may be useful for non-melanocytic skin cancers. It used to be the most common treatment of skin cancers, surgery being mostly reserved as a second-line of defence should radiotherapy fail. But gradually, over the years, as the long-term effects of radiation treatment began to be understood, and as surgical techniques advanced, surgery became the treatment of choice in the majority of cases.

Pregnancy

Women who have had a malignant melanoma may be advised not to become pregnant for about three years. This is not because pregnancy would increase their risk of metastasis, but simply to avoid additional stress during the period when recurrence most commonly occurs. Studies indicate that when treatment for skin cancer is necessary during pregnancy, it is as effective as at other times.

Surgery

Surgery may be the only possible choice of treatment in some cases, for example for carcinomas in the middle of the lower eyelid where radiotherapy would leave scarred tissue and reduce the protection given by the eyelid to the cornea.

As has already been stated, all melanomas should be removed surgically; most basal and squamous cell carcinomas in younger people are likely to be surgically excised, although those in awkward sites on the body may be treated with radiotherapy. However, the following may be treatment options for some carcinomas.

Details of the different surgical procedures are given in Chapter 6.

Curettage

Curettage is often done by dermatologists and by some family doctors. It is most suitable for lesions on the cheek, scalp, limbs and trunk of the body, and usually has acceptable cosmetic results.

After the injection of local anaesthetic, superficial basal cell carcinomas with a clearly defined margin can sometimes be simply scraped away using a spoon-shaped instrument called a curette. The tissue which has been removed should always be sent for histological examination (see p.34). Curettage may be followed by cautery to the base of the lesion. The treated area may then be left open to the air to promote healing; the scab which forms will fall off after two or three weeks, and the resulting scar will become less obvious with time. Even the thick scars which sometimes develop will gradually subside.

You may be asked to telephone your doctor's surgery after 10 to 14 days for the results of the histological examination. You will probably have to return for a check-up six to eight weeks after curettage, after which you may be able to keep a watch yourself for any further changes in the skin. If there is any cause for concern, however small, further check-ups may be necessary at regular intervals.

Mohs chemosurgery

Basal and squamous cell carcinomas can be removed by Mohs chemosurgery. This involves anaesthetising the skin, cutting out a circular section of malignant tissue, and looking at it under a microscope. Deeper slices of tissue are then removed in the same way, until microscopic examination reveals no further sign of malignant cells.

Although this procedure may leave quite a large scar, some doctors feel that it reduces the total amount of tissue which needs to be excised. It is useful for treating recurrent skin cancers, but apart from in the USA, where is has an established role in the treatment of skin cancer, it is not widely practised. It is a time-consuming and expensive procedure and in most cases has no apparent advantages over straightforward excision.

Cryosurgery

Cryosurgery is done using a local anaesthetic. It is a useful form of treatment for anyone who is unfit for surgery or unable to tolerate repeated radiotherapy sessions. It may be used to treat relatively superficial multiple lesions or a single large one as it avoids the need for extensive surgery and grafting. It can also be useful for squamous cell carcinomas of the ear as it does not destroy the cartilage. However, it does leave a scar.

Cryosurgery involves destroying the cancer by freezing it with liquid nitrogen or with an instrument called a cryoprobe. The tip of the cryoprobe is frozen and placed into the lesion to freeze the malignant tissue, which is then allowed to thaw for five to ten minutes. The tissue is then refrozen and covered with a dressing which remains in place for four to five weeks. During this time a weeping blister may form and the lesion will gradually die and may flake off, eventually leaving a scab which will drop off when the tissue has healed. A similar result can be obtained using liquid nitrogen to freeze the malignant tissue.

Cryosurgery, which freezes the tissue to a deep level, is distinct from the much more common procedure of cryotherapy, which only freezes the surface of tissue and which is sometimes used to remove actinic keratoses (see p.6) and very superficial basal cell carcinomas. Cryotherapy does not require any form of anaesthetic.

Radiotherapy

Surgery removes the cancer cells; radiotherapy destroys them. Surgery generally produces good cosmetic results, but radiotherapy may be more appropriate in some cases, for example for a carcinoma of the ear for which surgery would involve the removal of ear tissue. Radiotherapy may also be the treatment of choice for people for whom surgery is contraindicated, for example because of serious heart or breathing problems. It may sometimes also be useful in the treatment of skin carcinoma which has recurred despite repeated surgery.

Further details of radiotherapy are given in Chapter 9.

Adjuvant therapy

Chemotherapy and immunotherapy may be used in combination with surgery or radiotherapy for the treatment of advanced or metastatic disease. Details of these treatments are given in Chapter 10.

Clinical trials To be able to improve the treatment given for skin cancer, new drugs need to be tested and currently used drugs and radiotherapy regimes need to be tried in different ways. Therefore, people are sometimes asked to take part in clinical trials to compare a new treatment with an existing one.

If your doctor is involved in a trial of this sort, you may be asked if you would be willing to take part. The details of the trial will be explained to you, and you should make sure you fully understand what is entailed before you make a decision. You are under no obligation to agree to be involved, and if you refuse, the quality of the treatment you receive will not be affected in any way.

CHAPTER 4

Going in to hospital for an operation

The vast majority of smaller skin cancers can be removed during an out-patient appointment at a skin clinic or hospital. This chapter explains what may happen if you are admitted to hospital for surgical excision of a larger skin cancer, with or without the need for a graft or flap repair of the damaged skin.

You should receive a letter from the hospital telling you the date of your operation and any other details you need to know. Many hospitals also send out leaflets explaining their admission procedures and giving advice on what to take in with you. If you have been put on a shortlist and an operating slot becomes available unexpectedly, you may be telephoned and asked to come in at short notice, possibly within a day or two. Occasionally it is thought advisable to excise a skin cancer as soon as possible, in which case you may be admitted to hospital within a couple of days of your out-patient appointment.

Many skin cancers can be surgically excised using a local anaesthetic, often as day-case surgery (see below). Elderly or frail people, or those who have no one to care for them at home for a day or two after their operation, may remain in hospital overnight. Following straightforward excision and direct closure of the wound, you are unlikely to need to stay in hospital more than 24 hours. If you have a skin graft, you may be in hospital for four to five days, although some consultants are happy for their patients to go home after 48 hours. A skin graft on the leg is rather a different matter as the leg needs to be kept elevated and rested for a few days to allow the graft to heal, and in this case you may be in hospital for about a week.

At what time of the day you are admitted depends on the normal practice at your particular hospital. As a general guide, you may be admitted during the morning for an operation scheduled for the afternoon, or possibly during the previous afternoon or evening for one scheduled for the morning.

DAY-CASE SURGERY

Day-case surgery is being used increasingly for straightforward operations. It is likely to become even more common in the UK when the Government's proposed reduction in the number of hospital beds comes into effect. The average cost of an operation involving an overnight stay in hospital is considerably greater than the cost of the same operation done as a day case. Now that hospital expenditure is a major consideration, day-case surgery is seen as a sensible way of cutting costs and reducing the length of waiting lists.

You may be admitted to hospital for day-case surgery only an hour or two before your operation. If you have a local anaesthetic, you may be able to leave almost immediately after surgery, and within a few hours if you have a general anaesthetic.

Patients have to be screened very carefully by medical staff to make sure that only those whose general health is good, and who have appropriate home support when needed, are selected as day cases. Any necessary tests, such as a chest X-ray or electrocardiogram (ECG) can sometimes be done by a family doctor a week or two before your operation so that your time in hospital is kept to a minimum. Alternatively, pre-operative tests may be carried out at the out-patients' clinic so that your medical history, examination and investigation results can be collated by a hospital doctor before you enter hospital for your operation.

WHAT TO TAKE IN TO HOSPITAL

For day-case surgery you will only need something to read or otherwise occupy yourself during periods of waiting, and possibly slippers and a dressing gown (see below). If you are staying in hospital, the following list may be helpful.

1   *Nightclothes.* You will be given a hospital gown to wear during your operation. You will be able to dress again after day-case surgery, but if you are staying in hospital overnight, you should take your own nightclothes to put on when you are back on the ward.

2   *Slippers.* If you are being treated as an in-patient, you will need slippers to wear on the ward. Slippers may also be useful if you are having day-case surgery as you may walk from the day-case unit to the operating theatre, although you are more likely to be taken in a wheelchair or on a hospital trolley.

3   *Dressing gown.* You will need a dressing gown to wear on the ward as an in-patient, and may want to wear one over your hospital gown as you go to the operating theatre for day-case surgery.

4   *Towel and washing things.* You will need these if you are staying in hospital, and may also want to take them to have a wash before you leave after day-case surgery.

5   *Money.* A *small* amount of money may be useful for newspapers and the telephone. Large sums of money, wallets and handbags should not be taken into hospital as they may have to be kept in an unlocked cabinet by your bed. If you have to take any jewellery, valuables or large sums of money into hospital, they should be given to the ward sister for safe keeping when you are admitted. You will be given a receipt listing each item which you should keep

safe so that you can collect your possessions when you are discharged. However, hospital authorities strongly discourage people from bringing anything of great value with them unless absolutely necessary. It is better to make arrangements for any valuables you do not wish to leave at home to be looked after by a relative or friend while you are in hospital.

In some hospitals, there are lockers in the day-case unit, the key to which may be pinned to your operating gown.

6 *Books, magazines, puzzles, knitting.* There will inevitably be periods of waiting between visits from medical staff before your operation, and you may want something to occupy you during this time.

7 *Drugs you are already taking.* Once your admission has been arranged, your family doctor will have been asked to fill in a form stating all the drugs you are taking and their doses. You may also be asked to take your drugs with you when you are admitted to hospital so that their dosages can be checked and so that you can continue to be given any which are necessary. All your drugs will be kept for you during your stay as you must only take those which are given to you by medical staff. If you are asked to take your own drugs into hospital, they should be returned to you before you leave.

8 *Admission letter.* An admission letter will have been sent to you from the hospital, and you should take this with you when you are admitted for your operation.

Jewellery

As already mentioned, all jewellery should be left at home whenever possible to avoid it being lost or stolen. Wedding rings, or any other rings which are very precious to you or which cannot be removed, will be covered with adhesive tape before your operation as metal can cause electrical burns or electric shocks during the process of **diathermy** which is used to control bleeding during surgery.

HOSPITAL STAFF

The ward of a hospital is a busy place and can seem rather confusing and frightening. It may help to have an idea of the different medical staff you are likely to meet, and the jobs they do. The following details are based on current practice in the UK; the roles and titles of medical staff in other countries may differ slightly.

Nurses

The uniforms worn to distinguish nurses of different ranks will vary from hospital to hospital, but all nurses wear badges which state clearly their name and sometimes their grade. There are, of course, both male and female nurses, although women are still in the majority. The nursing grades are as follows.

1   The most senior nurse on the ward is the *ward sister* or *ward manager*. Each ward will have one ward sister who will be very experienced and able to answer any questions you may have. The ward sister has 24-hour a day responsibility for all the staff and patients on at least one ward, for the day-to-day running of the ward, standards of care etc., and is ultimately responsible for the ward even when not on duty. The ward sister will be a registered nurse (RN) or a registered general nurse (RGN), who has usually been qualified for at least five years. Ward sisters may wear a uniform of a single colour, often dark blue.

The male equivalent of the ward sister is a *charge nurse*, whose rank will be clearly displayed on his name badge. Charge nurses wear a white tunic.

2   When the ward sister is not on duty, there may be a *senior staff nurse* or a *team leader* of another grade in charge. The senior staff nurse is deputy to, and works closely with, the ward sister and, like her, this nurse will be very experienced.

3   Each ward may have several *staff nurses* – registered or registered general nurses who have completed their nursing training. They may be newly qualified or may have several years' experience, and will take charge of the ward when both the ward sister and senior staff nurse are unavailable. There are different grades of staff nurse, distinguished by different coloured belts, epaulettes, uniforms or, more rarely nowadays, hats.
     The more junior staff nurses are very often in their first or second post since qualifying. They are less involved in ward management, and are therefore able to work closely with the patients. Most of the staff nurses on a ward will be junior staff nurses.

4   *Enrolled nurses* are gradually being replaced and can now undergo a training programme to become staff nurses with the qualification of RGN. However, there are still many enrolled nurses working on hospital wards who are very experienced and sometimes team leaders (see above). They have undergone two years of training and, like the junior staff nurses, are mainly involved in patient care rather than ward management.

5   As student nurses now spend more time in college and less on the wards of hospitals, *health care assistants* (HCAs) are being brought in to take their place. These are unqualified nurses who have undergone six months' training on day release while working on a ward and who have then been assessed for a National Vocational Qualification (NVQ) by senior nurses. Health care assistants are able to carry out

all basic nursing duties except for the dispensing of drugs. They are supervised at all times by a qualified nurse.

6 The ward may also have several *nursing auxiliaries* who are present on the ward to deal with any non-medical jobs and to help with the basic care of patients such as making beds, serving tea, and putting away linen etc. Although nursing auxiliaries are not trained nurses, some are very experienced and have acquired greater responsibility.

7 Student nurses – *diploma nursing students* or Project 2000 *students* – are unpaid and allocated to the wards at various stages during their college-based training. They are mainly involved in observing and carrying out limited clinical tasks. In their last term before they qualify, they will be rostered on to nursing shifts and be part of a ward team.

Doctors

Each consultant surgeon in a hospital heads a team of doctors of different ranks, sometimes known as a 'firm'. You may meet some or all of them. These doctors can, of course, be men or women.

1 The *consultant surgeon* holds the ultimate responsibility for all the patients on the operating list, and for the work of all the staff in the 'firm'. Consultants have at least 10 to 15 years' experience as surgeons.

Unless you are being treated privately, you may not actually see the consultant surgeon who is responsible for your care, but should be visited on the ward before your operation by whichever surgeon is to perform it.

2 The *senior registrar* is a very experienced surgeon who has completed several years of training and will soon be appointed to a consultant post. This grade is soon to be phased out.

3 Your operation may be performed by a *registrar* rather than by a consultant surgeon or senior registrar. Registrars have trained as surgeons for at least two or three years and are able to carry out some surgery alone, assisting the consultant, or being assisted by the consultant, on more difficult operations.

4 Some hospitals employ *clinical assistants*, often very experienced surgeons who, for personal or family reasons, are not able to work full time, or family doctors with experience of surgery.

5 You may be examined before your operation by a *senior house officer* (SHO) or by a house surgeon (see below). Senior house officers have been qualified doctors for between one and five years, and are gaining further experience in hospital before becoming surgeons or specialising in another branch of medicine. They may perform some minor operations.

6 A *house surgeon* (or *house officer*) may be directly concerned with your care both before and after your operation, taking notes of your medical history and arranging for any necessary pre-operative investigations to be done, such as a blood count, chest X-ray or electrocardiogram. House officers are qualified doctors who have completed at least five years of undergraduate training and are working for a further year in hospital before becoming fully registered doctors. Although house officers do not perform surgery on their own, they may assist the surgeon in the operating theatre.

Anaesthetists are doctors who have trained in the administration of drugs which cause loss of sensation and/or consciousness (anaesthetics) and those which block feelings of pain (analgesics). If you are having a general anaesthetic, an anaesthetist may visit you before your operation to discuss any relevant details, such as any anaesthetics you have had in the past and any drugs you may be taking (see Chapter 5). This visit is not normally necessary for people having a local anaesthetic, which may be injected by the surgeon, although an anaesthetist will always be present throughout the operation.

Medical social workers

If any problems arise at home during your stay in hospital, or if you are concerned about being able to manage on your own once you return home, you can ask to talk to a medical social worker. Medical social workers work in close partnership with other medical staff in the hospital and will be able to give you advice and practical support. However, if your stay in hospital is short, and there is not enough time for you to see a medical social worker while you are there, an appointment may be made for someone to visit you at home. If necessary, you may be kept in hospital until nursing staff are happy that you will be able to manage at home or that arrangements have been made for you. 'Meals on wheels' or a home help should be available for anyone who needs them.

BEFORE THE OPERATION

Admission to the ward

When you arrive at the hospital, you should report to the main reception desk with your admission letter. The staff there will check your details and tell you which ward to go to. Once on the ward, the ward clerk or a nurse will deal with the clerical side of your admission, filling in the necessary forms with you. You will then be shown to your bed and told of any ward details such as meal times, where to find the toilets, day room etc.

In Britain, the 'Named Nurse Initiative' was introduced under the Government's Patients' Charter. Each patient in a National Health Service (NHS) hospital is allocated a *named nurse* who is responsible for planning that patient's nursing care throughout their stay. Your named nurse will admit you to the ward, look after you during your stay, and co-ordinate your discharge when the time comes. You will be allocated another nurse for other working shifts. The idea is for people to be identified as individuals who are known to at least one nurse on each shift and who are involved in their own care. The ward sister will, of course, still be informed of all aspects of your care, and will be able to discuss it with you or your relatives.

You may be asked to help your nurse draw up a care plan when you are admitted to the ward, and you should tell her of any ailments you have and of any preferences or dislikes, for example if you prefer to sleep with several pillows or if there are certain foods you do not want. Your nurse's name may be displayed above your bed or on your bedside locker so that your relatives and other nursing and medical staff know who to talk to about your care. Your care plan may be kept at the bottom of your bed, but wherever it is, it is available for you to read. Nursing staff may tick off a checklist as they carry out the various procedures and will update the care plan with you as the need arises.

Several pre-operative tests need to be done to make sure you are fit for surgery. The nurse will measure your blood pressure, temperature and pulse. A sample of your urine may be taken for analysis to make sure you do not have diabetes or any disorder of the kidneys which could complicate the operation. You may also be weighed as the anaesthetist may need to know your weight in order to be able to calculate the dose of anaesthetic you require.

When your discharge is planned, the nursing staff will need to be sure that someone will be able to collect you and take you home when the time comes. If this is not possible, hospital transport may be arranged for you. If you are due to go home the day after your operation, the nurses will have to be sure you can manage. The effects of general anaesthetic gases, and other agents used by the anaesthetist, can stay in your body for several days, and although you may feel you are fully recovered, your reaction times will be slow and you may continue to feel sick and light-headed for at least a day or two.

Do tell a nurse if you have any problems or if you are anxious about *any* aspect of your hospital stay.

Anti-embolism stockings

Once you are settled on the ward, a nurse may measure your legs for anti-embolism stockings (often called TEDS – **t**hromboembolic **d**eterrent **s**tockings) to wear during your operation and until you are mobile afterwards. The stockings help prevent blood clots (**thrombi**) forming in the veins deep within the legs by improving the return of venous blood to the heart. They are used routinely in some hospitals. Although they may feel uncomfortable, particularly when the weather is hot, there is no doubt as to their value.

The normal activity of the muscles in the legs helps to keep the blood moving through them. During long periods of bed rest or anaesthesia, these muscles are inactive and the circulation of blood in the legs slows down. A blood clot (**thrombus**) is thus more likely to form which can block the passage of blood through the vein, causing **thrombosis**. If a piece of this clot break off, it forms an **embolus** which, if it travels through the circulation and lodges in a vital organ such as the lung, can cause **pulmonary embolism**, with serious consequences.

The nurse will measure your calf and thigh and the length of your leg, and will give you a pair of stockings of the correct size. If you have a history of varicose veins or thrombosis which increases your risk of developing a blood clot, you will probably have to wear the stockings throughout your hospital stay. Otherwise you will probably not need to put them on until you are preparing to go to the operating theatre. You will be told to keep them on until you are up and about again after your operation. Anti-embolism stockings are not normally necessary for people having local anaesthesia or very brief operations.

Heparin injections

Anyone with a previous history of thrombosis, or otherwise at high risk of developing blood clots, may be given heparin injections during their stay in hospital. Heparin is an anticoagulant which occurs naturally in the body, thinning the blood and preventing it from clotting.

Visit by a doctor

As has already been mentioned, a house surgeon or senior house officer will visit you on the ward before your operation to take details of your medical history – including any allergies you may have and any drugs you are taking – and to examine you. Your family doctor may have already filled in a form giving the names and dosages of any drugs you have been prescribed, and you should have been told what to do about these. Do not forget to tell the hospital doctor of any other drugs you have been taking which your family doctor may not be aware of, such as vitamin supplements, cough medicines, aspirins etc., which are available from a pharmacy without the need for prescription.

If you normally take a contraceptive pill or hormone replacement tablets, you may have been told to stop these for a time before your operation. If you are still taking them when you enter hospital, for example if you have been called for your operation at short notice, you should tell the doctor. Modern contraceptive pills contain much lower doses of hormones than the earlier ones, but they are still sometimes associated with complications from blood clots. Although the risks are much lower with the newer pills, some surgeons still prefer their patients to stop taking them for at least a month before surgery.

A medical examination will be carried out to identify any illness or infection you may have which could complicate the use of a general anaesthetic. If you are over 50 years of age or a heavy smoker, you may have to have a chest X-ray and an electrocardiogram so that any potential anaesthetic complications due to breathing or heart problems can be picked up.

Consent forms

You will be asked to sign a consent form declaring that your operation has been explained to you and that you understand what it entails and have agreed to it taking place. You are also giving your permission for the doctors to take whatever action they feel to be appropriate should some emergency occur during surgery, and for any necessary anaesthetic to be given to you. Do read this form carefully, and ask the doctor to explain anything you do not understand.

Visit by the surgeon

The surgeon who is to perform your operation may also visit you on the ward to check that all is well and to identify the area of your skin cancer, and possibly mark it with an indelible felt-tip pen if it is not obvious.

Visit by the anaesthetist

The anaesthetist will probably come to see you to ask you about anything that may be relevant to the choice of anaesthetic given to you, about any anaesthetics you have had before, any drugs you are taking, and about your general health. It is important that you answer these questions as fully as possible so that you are given the anaesthetic which is safest for you. If you have had any problems in the past such as an allergy to a particular anaesthetic, it will be helpful if you know the name of the drug concerned or the hospital where the operation was carried out. The appropriate records can then be checked to make sure another type of anaesthetic is used. You should also tell the anaesthetist if you know of any other member of your family who has reacted against a particular drug, as you may have the same problem.

The anaesthetist may also want to examine you and to look at the result of any tests you have had.

Anaesthetics have improved considerably during the last few years, and a pre-medication ('pre-med.') is now not always given routinely. If you or your anaesthetist feel that you are very anxious and need something to relax you, you may be given a pre-med., a sedative given by mouth or injection, two or three hours before surgery. If you enter hospital the day before your operation and think that you will be too anxious to sleep that night, you can ask the house surgeon or senior house officer for something to help you.

Do talk to the anaesthetist about any problems or worries you have concerning your anaesthesia.

False teeth

The anaesthetist will examine your mouth and teeth. If you have any false teeth or dental bridges, you should tell the anaesthetist as these will have to be removed before you go into the operating theatre. A broken or loose tooth can be inhaled into the lungs during surgery. You should also point out any teeth which are crowned. At some hospitals you will be able to wear your false teeth until you reach the operating theatre rather than having to take them out in the ward.

'Nil by mouth'

This is a term which means that neither food nor drink must be swallowed. In order to prevent vomiting and the risk of choking on your vomit while you are anaesthetised, you will be told not to eat or drink anything for four to six hours before an operation done using a general anaesthetic, although you will be able to have a few sips of water with any tablets you need to take. If you are admitted the night before surgery, you will be able to have supper on the ward. If you enter hospital in the morning and your operation is to be that afternoon, you should not eat or drink for about six hours beforehand, although some anaesthetists now allow their patients to drink clear fluids up to three hours pre-operatively.

Smoking

If you are a heavy smoker and have not been able to cut down or stop altogether, you will be advised not to smoke in the hours before your operation. It is, of course, much better to stop smoking some months before surgery. The carbon monoxide contained in cigarette smoke poisons the blood by replacing some of the oxygen which is carried in it and which is vital to processes such as wound healing. The nicotine in cigarettes reduces the blood supply by constricting the blood vessels.

Obesity

Obesity adds to the risk of general anaesthesia, and for this reason people who are very overweight should try to lose weight before entering hospital. Some surgeons are reluctant to carry out non-emergency operations on heavy smokers or obese patients as they consider the risks to be too great. However, starting a long, strict diet before your operation may also be inadvisable. The consultant will have assessed your weight when seeing you at your out-patients appointment, and will probably have given you some guidance at that time.

Waiting

It may seem that you have been admitted to hospital unnecessarily early, and you may have to wait on the ward with little to do. Apart from having to be seen by all the medical staff mentioned above, who are responsible for many other patients as well, time will also have been allowed for the assessment of any medical problems you may have, and for the results of any blood tests to be received.

Sometimes operations have to be cancelled at the last moment if an emergency has arisen or an earlier operation has taken longer than expected. Although this would be distressing, and may be awkward for someone who has had to arrange child care or time off work, it would only occur if an operation taking place before your own had met with complications or an emergency case had been admitted. If this does occur, you may be sent home and called again at the earliest opportunity. Do try not to get upset. Other operations taking place on the same day may be more urgent than yours and cannot be postponed. Under the terms of the Patients' Charter, a cancelled operation must be done within one month.

As surgery done before yours may take longer than expected, you will probably be given only an approximate time for your operation, being told if it is scheduled for the morning or afternoon.

Leaving the ward for your operation

Before being taken from the ward to the anaesthetic room or operating theatre, you will be given a hospital operating gown to wear, and a plastic-covered bracelet bearing your name and an identifying hospital number will be attached to one or both of your wrists. If you are having a general anaesthetic, you will then be taken from the ward on a hospital trolley. If you are having a local anaesthetic, you may be able to walk to the operating room, but are more likely to be taken in a wheelchair or on a trolley.

The anaesthetic room

In the anaesthetic room, a small tube called a **cannula** will be inserted into a vein in the back of your hand. The cannula will be kept in place throughout the operation and provides a channel for the administration of drugs. Cannulas are often inserted routinely whatever type of anaesthetic is being used.

Sometimes anaesthetics are administered in the operating theatre itself, and this is certainly likely to be the case for the injection of a local anaesthetic.

Once the anaesthetic has taken effect, which will happen within seconds, you are ready for your operation.

CHAPTER 5

Anaesthesia for surgery

The injection of local anaesthetic is relatively simple and straightforward and needs little explanation. Therefore most of the information in this chapter concerns the use of general anaesthetics.

LOCAL ANAESTHESIA

Many small skin cancers can be surgically removed using local anaesthesia. A local anaesthetic is a drug which blocks the sensation of pain in the area of the body into which it is injected. It has the advantage of allowing you to be awake during surgery and to be able to get up and move around immediately afterwards. It does not cause post-operative nausea or drowsiness. The anaesthetic may sting as it enters your body, and some people do find the injection painful. Although you are likely to be able to sense touch once the anaesthetic has taken effect, you should tell the doctor if you feel any pain as you may require more anaesthetic drug.

Spinal and epidural anaesthesia

These are types of regional local anaesthesia in which the anaesthetic drug is injected between the vertebrae of the spine into the space around the nerves in the back. Spinal and epidural anaesthetics cause numbness in the legs and groin which lasts for three to five hours. They therefore give effective post-operative pain relief for a period, and are sometimes used for operations to remove skin cancers in the legs or lower body.

The two types of anaesthesia are similar, but a spinal anaesthetic will temporarily cause more weakness in the legs, and thus reduce the need for other local anaesthetic drugs.

You may be given a sedative with a spinal or epidural anaesthetic if you do not wish to be awake throughout your operation. Do ask the anaesthetist about this if you are concerned.

Once the anaesthetic has been injected into your back, it will take effect after five to ten minutes and your legs and lower body will become numb and heavy.

Brachial/axillary plexus block

This is another type of regional local anaesthetic which can be used for the surgical removal of a skin cancer on the arm. The anaesthetic is injected at the top of the arm, usually in the armpit (axillary) but sometimes into the shoulder (supra-clavicular), and anaesthetises the collection of nerves supplying the whole of the arm.

Nerve block

A nerve block involves the injection of local anaesthetic around a nerve, possibly a short distance from the site of the skin cancer. The nerves follow a predictable path through the body and there are several sites at which they can be conveniently blocked.

GENERAL ANAESTHESIA

A general anaesthetic will put you to sleep so that you have no feeling in any part of your body. It may be an **intravenous anaesthetic**, injected into a vein in your hand or arm through a plastic tube, or an **inhalational anaesthetic** in the form of a gas which you breathe in. In fact, both types are normally used, although you will usually only be aware of the injection which sends you off to sleep. An advantage of general anaesthesia is that you will be in a deep sleep throughout the operation and will not move or otherwise interrupt the work of the surgeon.

Risks of general anaesthesia

People with certain medical conditions, such as serious heart or lung disease, may not be given general anaesthetics as they are potentially at greater risk.

Some people are afraid of being put to sleep by a general anaesthetic, but the risk is small. In Britain, approximately 3 people in every 500 000 undergoing an operation under general anaesthesia die as a direct result of the anaesthetic. This risk is low when compared to the number of deaths which occur, for example, as a result of road accidents, but it has to be borne in mind. If you are worried about it, do discuss it with the anaesthetist.

The risk involved in the use of local anaesthetics is even lower.

Other medication

The anaesthetist will explain about other tablets and drugs which may be required before the operation. You may be given the option of having a 'pre-med.' (see p.53), sometimes in the form of tablets or a syrup, but usually as an injection given one to two hours before the operation. If you are anxious about your operation, you may wish to ask for a 'pre-med.' if their use is not routine in your hospital.

If there is a reason for you to have antibiotics or blood-thinning drugs, this will also be explained to you. You may be given any drugs which you normally take, such as diuretics ('water tablets') or drugs to reduce high blood pressure.

Before your operation

If you are having a general anaesthetic, you will probably be told not to have anything to eat or drink for at least six hours before the operation ('nil by mouth', see p.54), although you may be able to drink clear fluids up to three or four hours pre-operatively.

If you are having a 'pre-med.', it may be given to you while you are still on the ward, and you will soon begin to feel sleepy. There is no need to be alarmed: the 'pre-med.' is not an anaesthetic in itself, it is only to relax you so that you are not anxious before the operation.

When the time comes to take you to the operating theatre, you will be asked several questions to confirm your identity and to make sure that you are ready for the operation. These questions may be repeated several times by different people: many people have many types of operations each day in a hospital and checks are essential to avoid mistakes.

When you are taken from the ward, you may go to the anaesthetic room or straight to the operating theatre to be given your anaesthetic. The anaesthetist, or an assistant, will fit monitoring devices to watch over you while you are asleep. These may include a little probe which goes on your finger to measure the amount of oxygen in your blood, an electrocardiogram (ECG) to measure your heart beat, and a cuff around your arm to measure your blood pressure. Once the anaesthetist is happy with the readings from these monitors, the anaesthesia will start.

The anaesthetist will remain with you throughout the operation to make sure you are asleep and that the function of your heart and lungs is satisfactory. Once the anaesthetic has been injected into the tube in your hand or arm, you will fall asleep within seconds. The drug which makes you go to sleep may sting a little as it enters the vein from the cannula, but this feeling does not last long.

Several different types of drugs will be given to you during your operation:

* *induction agents* to bring on sleep;
* *maintenance agents* to keep you asleep;
* *analgesics* to stop you feeling pain after the operation;
* *anti-emetics* to help stop you feeling sick after the operation.

Local anaesthetic will probably be injected into the wound at the site of removal of the skin cancer during surgery, so you should have little or no pain when you wake up.

When the operation is over, the anaesthetist will stop giving you the drugs that were keeping you asleep, and you will probably be taken to a recovery room or step-down ward.

The recovery room

The nurses in the recovery room are specially trained to care for patients coming round from anaesthetics after an operation. You will stay in this room, still watched over by monitoring equipment, until you are fully awake and ready to be returned to your own ward.

If you are in any pain when you wake up, the staff in the recovery room will be able to give you something to relieve it. This can be an injection, either through the cannula which was used to put you to sleep or into your arm or leg, although often tablets such as paracetamol or aspirin will be enough.

The step-down ward

If you are going home on the same day as your operation, you may be taken to a step-down ward. The nurses on this ward will make sure that you are fit to go home and that your journey will be safe and pain free. They will also want to be sure that you have a responsible adult to care for you once you are at home.

Back on the ward

If you are not going home the same day, you will be taken back to your own ward, where the anaesthetist may visit you to ensure that you are having adequate pain relief and have no ill-effects from your operation. Do tell the anaesthetist if you have any concerns or questions.

Side-effects of general anaesthesia

There are some side-effects related to the use of anaesthetics, but these are usually minor and do not last very long. The most common are nausea and vomiting. You may have a sore throat after your operation, possibly due to the 'dry' anaesthetic gases used to keep you asleep during surgery, or to the tube which may have been used to help you to breathe. Whatever the reason, any soreness usually disappears after two or three days and can be eased by the use of simple painkillers.

PAIN RELIEF

The house surgeon, senior house officer or nurses on your ward will be able to give you analgesics if you have any pain. However, if these are not enough, do tell the anaesthetist or ward staff who may be able to give you something more effective.

The amount of discomfort suffered after any operation varies from person to person, and of course depends on the extent of the surgery involved. Some people have only slight discomfort for 12 to 24 hours, whereas others may need pain-killing injections for a day or two.

The operations

The surgical treatment of all skin cancers involves excision of the malignant lesion itself together with a surrounding margin of normal-looking tissue. What happens once the cancer has been excised depends largely on its size and site and on whether surgical reconstruction is necessary. After excision of a small lesion, the skin may simply be reclosed by suturing, whereas reconstruction of the area by skin grafts or flaps may be needed following the removal of a larger one.

EXCISION AND DIRECT CLOSURE

The size of the margin of apparently normal tissue removed will depend on the type of skin cancer and its clinical appearance. Nodular or cystic basal cell carcinomas, which have well-defined edges and tend not to be diffusely invasive, can sometimes be excised with a margin of only a few millimetres. Squamous cell carcinomas, on the other hand, tend to be more diffuse and a margin of at least 1 cm of apparently normal tissue may need to be removed with them. All malignant melanomas and some of the more diffuse basal cell carcinomas, such as the morphoeic type, must be excised with a wide margin, the actual extent of which depends on the depth of invasion of the malignant tissue.

The area to be excised may already have been marked with a felt-tip pen or this may be done in the operating theatre. An incision will be made along the line drawn around the lesion and a block of tissue will be excised and sent for subsequent histological examination. Direct closure of the wound leaves a

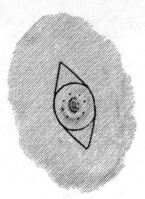

Surgical excision. The dots mark out the skin cancer; the solid lines encircle the margin of normal tissue which will need to be excised to obtain a good cosmetic result, for example on the temple beside the eye.

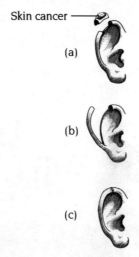

Skin cancer ⟶

(a)

(b)

(c)

Rim advancement. An example of a flap repair, used here following excision of a small lesion from the rim of the ear (a). The lower part of the remaining rim is separated from the ear lobe (b), advanced to close the defect, and stitched in place (c). Some shortening of the ear lobe is inevitable.

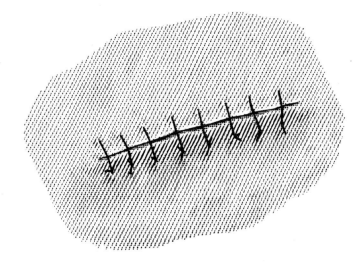

Sutures. Interrupted stitches like these may be used to close the incision following surgical excision of a skin cancer.

linear scar and, whenever possible, the incision is made along a natural crease line in the skin to help hide the scar. The type of sutures used will depend on the site of the lesion and on the personal preference of the surgeon. Small, interrupted stitches may be made with a non-absorbable material which will need to be removed after a few days. Alternatively, a continuous suture may be made beneath the skin with either absorbable (dissolving) or non-absorbable suture material.

SKIN GRAFTS

A skin graft is a piece of skin which has been detached from its own blood supply and transferred to another site. Skin may be grafted to repair a wound made during excision of a skin lesion

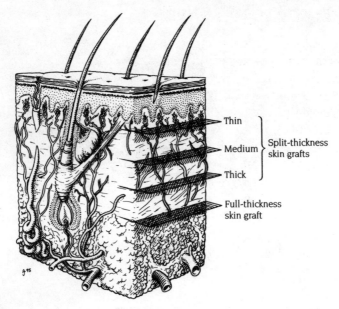

Thin

Medium } Split-thickness skin grafts

Thick

Full-thickness skin graft

Skin grafts. This diagram shows the depths of skin removed from a donor site for different split-thickness and full-thickness skin grafts.

when direct closure is not possible. Grafting may be done immediately after excision or a day or two later, depending on the surgeon's preferred practice and on the general health of the patient.

The skin graft may need to be secured at the recipient site with stitches, glue or staples, or it may simply be covered with a dressing. The recipient site must have an adequate blood supply to enable the graft to 'take', i.e. to reattach and reform its blood vessels.

The donor site is selected on the basis of a good match of skin colour, texture and distribution of hair, to obtain as thick a graft as possible without damaging the donor site, and to be as inconspicuous as possible when it has healed.

Split-thickness skin grafts

Also known as partial thickness grafts, these can be thin, intermediate or thick, depending on the amount of dermis taken from the donor site. They do have some limitations in that skin from a distant site may be of a different colour from that at the recipient site. They also have a tendency to contract and thus to distort adjacent structures and they are therefore not suitable for use in areas around orifices such as the eyes, mouth and nose. But there are several advantages to split-thickness skin grafting: large donor sites are available which allow large areas of skin to be replaced; the grafted skin will not be rejected as it has been taken from the same individual; and a donor site is selected which will heal spontaneously without scarring, although it may remain slightly discoloured.

Full-thickness skin grafts

For relatively shallow defects and where better colour match and contour correction are desired, full-thickness skin grafts may be used. A segment of skin is removed from the donor site which includes the epidermis and the entire dermis. These grafts are most useful following excision of skin cancers in the head and neck, when small pieces of replacement tissue are required. The donor skin is often taken from in front of or behind the ear or from the neck.

The disadvantages of full-thickness skin grafts are that they leave a scar at the donor site, and are slightly more prone to failure to take than split-thickness grafts. The limited area of donor skin available for a full-thickness graft makes it unsuitable for the repair of large areas of skin.

Full-thickness grafts can include other tissues, such as fat or cartilage, when these are required for reconstruction, for example of the nose. They are then known as **composite grafts**.

SKIN FLAPS

In some cases, local skin flaps may be more appropriate than skin grafts. A flap is a segment of tissue which has been cut away and moved to a nearby recipient site, but which remains attached to its original site by a pedicle of skin (or subcutaneous tissue) which carries the blood supply. Survival of the flap is dependent on keeping the blood supply and lymphatic drainage within its pedicle intact and functioning. Thus, unlike a graft, a flap keeps at least part of its original blood supply.

A flap may be made up of skin, muscle, fat and bone. It is a useful means of replacing a bulk of tissue which has been excised with a more deep-rooted skin cancer. The skin and soft tissue of a skin flap will match that in the adjacent recipient site in colour and texture, and enough depth of tissue can be transferred to repair any contour deformity. Tissue is removed from the donor site in such a way that scars can often be hidden in skin creases. Occasionally, for better contouring of the tissue, a flap repair requires two operations a few weeks apart to allow the flap to heal in before dividing the pedicle.

Free flaps

A free flap, or **microvascular flap**, is a flap of skin which has been completely removed from the donor site and reattached at the recipient site by rejoining its blood vessels to those in the recipient site using very fine microsurgical instruments and high-powered magnification.

Free flaps may be used to repair large defects, following more radical surgery for neglected or recurrent skin cancers, or to replace specialised tissue such as bone.

LYMPH NODE EXCISION

In the past, when a malignant melanoma was excised, lymph

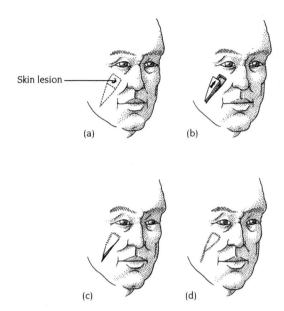

Skin lesion

(a)

(b)

(c)

(d)

An example of a skin flap. (a) The skin lesion is excised together with a square of surrounding normal tissue. A triangular flap of tissue (b) is then repositioned to fill in the defect (c), and the narrower part of the V shape is closed by stitching (d).

nodes in the area around it were sometimes removed routinely. Now that diagnosis is normally made before metastasis occurs, routine lymph node excision is no longer considered to be necessary. However, if it is suspected that a skin cancer has spread to the lymph nodes, or when a lesion is very close to a lymph node field, the nodes may be excised, either at the same time as the skin cancer is removed or at a later date.

CHAPTER 7

After your operation

IN HOSPITAL

What happens after your operation will depend on whether you have had a simple excision of a lesion and direct closure of the wound, a skin graft or flap repair, and on the site of the lesion, your general state of health and the normal practice of your particular surgeon.

In general, you may be able to go home almost immediately after day-case surgery involving a local anaesthetic, or at most after an hour or two. If you have had a general anaesthetic, you will probably have to wait a little longer until its immediate effects have worn off and you are fit to travel. You should not drive yourself home, however well you feel. Most types of car insurance do not cover people to drive for at least 48 hours after a general anaesthetic, and there is always a risk that you may feel a bit weak for a while after any type of anaesthesia. If you do not have a friend or family member who can collect you from hospital, it may be possible for transport to be arranged for you, but do mention this before your operation, preferably before you enter hospital, to allow time for arrangements to be made.

If you are staying in hospital overnight, you will be returned to your ward when you come round from the anaesthetic. Some people feel quite well and able to eat as soon as they wake up, but others feel drowsy for the rest of the day and possibly quite sick and light headed for a few hours at least. If your mouth is dry, you can take sips of water, but drinking too much immediately after your operation can make any nausea worse. You will be able to eat as soon as you want to as your digestive system will not have been affected by the surgery.

After excision and direct closure

Little aftercare is required following straightforward excision of a skin cancer and direct closure of the wound. The wound must be kept clean and dry for at least 24 to 48 hours, after which, if it is healing satisfactorily, epithelium will have grown over it. Provided you take sensible precautions not to irritate any stitches, no special care is needed after this. The specific advice you are given will depend on the site and size of the excision and on the normal practice of your surgeon.

After a skin graft or flap repair

Drips
If you have had a large area of skin grafted or a flap repair, there may be a drip in your arm when you regain consciousness after surgery. The drip contains a specially balanced solution to replace the fluids which have been lost from your body during the operation. Drips are sometimes left in overnight, but may be removed after a couple of hours or so once you are able to drink freely. They are also occasionally used following excision and direct closure of a wound.

Drainage tubes
If you have had a flap repair, there may be a small tube extending out of the side of the wound dressing, possibly draining into a bag or bottle. Drainage tubes are inserted to allow any excess fluid or blood to drain away from the wound, and they may be held in place with a stitch. They will be removed when leakage from the wound stops, usually within 48 hours at most.

Grafting skin on the ward

Skin is usually grafted in the operating theatre immediately after a lesion has been excised, but sometimes although it is removed from the donor site during surgery it is not grafted until a day or so later, when the recipient site has cleared of blood and fluid. (Skin can be kept for up to three weeks, refrigerated in a special glass container.) A nurse or doctor on the ward will measure the operation site, cut the skin to the size required and lay it carefully in place. The graft may then be left exposed or covered with a protective dressing to prevent it rubbing on your clothes or bedclothes.

Wound dressings

Skin grafts require more post-operative care than wounds which have been closed by stitches following excision. The dressing over a full-thickness or split-thickness skin graft will be left in place for four to seven days, and should not be interfered with while the skin heals unless absolutely necessary. Even if the graft has taken by the time the first dressing is removed, another protective dressing will be needed for a further week or more until the skin has become more firmly attached and resilient. Protective dressings will have to be changed periodically at the hospital or by the practice nurse at your doctor's surgery. If you are unable to get to the surgery, arrangements can be made for a district nurse to visit you at home.

Care of a skin graft

The skin graft and the donor site will be red and raw looking, and you may be quite shocked when you first see them. But they will change over the following weeks and months and, although the skin will always remain scarred, it will eventually become much paler in colour and more normal in appearance. The grafted skin should not be washed until it has healed completely.

Grafted skin tends to become dry as it has fewer sweat and sebaceous glands than the skin it replaces, and its circulation will not be as good. Therefore, once you no longer need a dressing, you should gently massage an oily cream into the graft, twice a day for at least six months, to help keep it moist and supple. Perfumed oils and creams are not suitable for this purpose, as they could irritate the skin.

Grafted skin is more susceptible to sunburn in the first six months and you should therefore always use a *complete sunblock* to protect it from sun exposure. Care should also be taken to avoid damage by heat or cold.

Care of the donor site

Skin for grafting is usually taken from the top of the legs or arms. Wherever the donor site is, it will also need some care, and may be more uncomfortable than the graft itself. It will be raw and graze like for a while, but the skin usually heals spontaneously as the dermis becomes covered with epithelium. The donor site should be kept dry and, unless instructed otherwise, you should not bath or shower until it has healed. It may be covered with a thin layer of gauze with a dressing on top to absorb any leakage of fluid or blood. The dressing may be transparent so that the wound can be inspected easily, and it will be kept in place for 10 to 14 days while the skin grows back. It may become quite stained during this time, but should not be interfered with until the skin has healed and cannot easily be pulled away. A mildly unpleasant odour is common but if it is offensive or accompanied by a raised body temperature, it can be a sign of infection.

Once the skin on the donor site has healed, the dressing may be soaked off in a bath, but if your clothes or bedclothes rub the new skin, you may need a new dressing to protect it. The skin should then be massaged daily using an unperfumed oily cream (see above).

Immobilisation

The part of your body onto which skin has been grafted will have to be kept immobilised for some time to allow the graft to heal. If you have had a skin graft on your face, you should avoid bending or putting your head down for at least 48 hours to prevent blood rushing to the wound and destabilising the graft. If you have had a graft on your arm, you may be given a sling to prevent you moving it.

A leg which has had a skin graft must be rested and elevated to reduce swelling and prevent the pressure of blood in its veins from rupturing the small, newly connecting blood vessels. A plaster of Paris cast (a 'back slab') may be fitted over the back of your lower leg and held in place with bandages to provide support and to stop you moving your foot. How long you need to remain immobile depends on the site and size of the operation, but you may have to rest in hospital for up to one week.

Until you are able to move around freely again, you may be given injections of heparin or a similar blood-thinning drug daily or twice daily to help prevent blood clots developing (see p.51).

A day or two after the graft has taken, you will be able to get up and walk to the bathroom with the assistance of a nurse. You will feel quite weak and unsteady to begin with, but will gradually be able to increase the amount of exercise you can do. You will have to wear an elastic 'Tubigrip' bandage on your leg during the day for 6 to 12 weeks at least, but should always take it off at night. When sitting, your leg should be raised to prevent blood and fluid collecting and causing it to swell.

Painkillers

Regular pain-killing tablets should ease any discomfort, and are only likely to be necessary for 48 hours after surgery. You may be given pain-killing injections while in hospital if tablets are not effective. Injections may also be given to anyone who is vomiting and will probably incorporate an anti-emetic to lessen the sickness.

Physiotherapy

You may be visited on the ward by a physiotherapist who will advise you of any exercises you should do to assist your blood circulation while you are immobile. You may also need to do deep-breathing exercises to help avoid chest infection, particularly if you have respiratory problems or are a smoker.

Going home

Before you go home, the hospital staff must be satisfied that you will be able to manage. For example, you may need to move your bed downstairs and have a temporary toilet arrangement if your mobility is reduced. If necessary, a medical social worker (see p.48) will visit you on the ward to discuss the help available through the social services, such as 'meals on wheels' or a home help, and to make arrangements for when you leave hospital. Do discuss any potential problems with nursing staff before you leave hospital so that the social services can be alerted in good time if necessary.

When you are discharged from hospital, you may be given a letter to take to your family doctor or it may be sent directly to him or her by the hospital. This discharge letter will give your doctor all the relevant information about your operation and any follow-up treatment you require.

AT HOME

Following simple excision and wound closure, there is little you will need to do to take care of your wound once you are at home. Stitches which are made of a non-absorbable material will probably have to be removed at your doctor's surgery.

However, after a skin graft on your leg, you will have to take things easy, gradually increasing the amount you are able to do comfortably each day. You will be able to walk and take gentle exercise, but will feel very tired if you overdo it to begin with. Do not stand for long periods as this causes the blood to pool in your legs and can lead to problems with the grafted skin, and certainly to swelling and discomfort. When sitting, always keep your leg raised, preferably with your heel level with your heart, to reduce swelling. Try to sit to prepare food and do the washing up etc. or, better still, get some help with these chores for a few weeks. Ask your doctor's advice before you start driving again.

If you still have a dressing on a skin graft, it will have to be changed regularly, possibly as often as every other day if on the leg. This can be done by the practice nurse at your doctor's surgery, or by a district nurse at your home if it is difficult for you to get there.

FOLLOW-UP EXAMINATIONS

However straightforward your operation, you will probably be given an appointment to attend a dressing clinic or out-patients department a week or two later for a check-up and to receive the results of the histological examination of the tissue removed. Following a skin graft or flap repair, you may also have to return for a check-up about three months after surgery to make sure that all is well.

It is important that regular follow-up examinations are done, for at least the first two or three years after surgery for a malignant melanoma, until the risk of recurrence has reduced. The intervals between your follow-up appointments will depend on the routine practice of your doctor and on the risk associated with your particular type of skin cancer. With malignant melanoma, about 80 per cent of metastases become apparent within two years of treatment, 90 per cent within five years, and almost all within ten years. After ten years, life expectancy returns to that of the general population.

CHAPTER 8

Possible complications of surgery

There can be complications following any type of surgery or general anaesthesia. Although minor complications are not uncommon, serious ones are rare. Some are related to an underlying health problem rather than to the operation itself, but the majority of people whose skin cancers are removed by a dermatologist or surgeon will not experience any problems. The general complications described in this chapter can occasionally occur following surgery for larger cancers and/or reconstructive surgery by means of skin grafts or flaps.

IMMEDIATE COMPLICATIONS

Chest infection

Chest infection is possible after general anaesthesia for any type of operation, particularly if a painful wound makes breathing difficult. Chest infections are more common amongst smokers and when mobility is restricted after surgery. It is important to keep the lungs well aerated after your operation and, if necessary, you will be shown how to do some deep-breathing exercises before you leave hospital.

Deep vein thrombosis

When possible, you will be given anti-embolism stockings to wear if your mobility is reduced post-operatively (see p.50). These exert a graded pressure along the length of the leg and thereby assist the circulation of blood through it, reducing the risk of blood clots. Raising your legs when sitting will also help to reduce the risk of thrombosis.

If you are thought to be at risk of deep vein thrombosis, you will be given a course of blood-thinning drugs while in hospital. Medical advice should be sought immediately if you experience pain, swelling or inflammation of the leg as these may be signs of a blood clot.

Pulmonary embolism

Pulmonary embolism arises secondary to a blood clot else-where, particularly in the legs, and can be life threatening (see p.50). Should you develop a deep vein thrombosis, you will be given heparin or warfarin to reduce the risk of pulmonary embolism. The signs of pulmonary embolism are shortness of breath and/or pain on breathing, for which immediate medical advice should be sought

Pain and bruising

Some discomfort in the wound is normal after any operation, but it is unusual to have severe pain which cannot be controlled by the regular use of painkillers such as paracetamol or aspirin. Local anaesthetic is often injected into the wound before it is closed, and this will help to reduce any pain in the first few post-operative hours. However, some people may need pain-killing injections for a day or so post-operatively.

If pain persists after a few days, it may be a sign that a wound infection is developing, and you should seek medical advice.

Even minor operations can cause bruising which may be severe and can last for several days or weeks. A bruise may not become apparent until some time after surgery, and its appearance may be quite distressing. However, even when severe it is unlikely to be a cause for concern.

Haematoma

A haematoma is a collection of blood which has leaked from the tissues during or after an operation. Sometimes blood which is unable to escape may collect under a skin flap. Although haematomas usually resolve spontaneously, they can be painful and cause quite severe bruising.

Pyrexia

Pyrexia is simply fever which can occur in the first 24 hours after surgery. Persistent fever should be investigated as it can be a sign of infection or deep vein thrombosis.

Wound infection

Infection will cause the wound to become red, hard and tender to the touch. It may also make you feel generally unwell, possibly with a fever and sweating.

If pus from a wound collects in an **abscess**, it will become red, hard and tender. The pus will have to be released and you may need a course of antibiotics to prevent systemic infection. Very rarely, severe infection such as gas gangrene can occur which will require immediate treatment in hospital.

Fluid collection

A skin flap may become raised by a collection of fluid which forms a **seroma** beneath it. The fluid is usually a light golden colour, not bloody, and probably comes from the lymphatics. In some cases it may have to be drawn off through a needle inserted into the scar, which is a painless procedure but which may need to be repeated.

LATE COMPLICATIONS

Any late complications are likely to relate to the appearance of the scar, such as thickening or the development of excessive pigmentation (**hyperpigmentation**). Contracture of a graft may pull or distort adjacent structures, for example the eyelid. Contracture of a full-thickness graft can cause it to become elevated and swollen, known as the **pin cushion effect**. This usually settles with time and massage, but occasionally requires revisionary surgery. Flaps may be similarly affected.

Large excisions, particularly in the limbs, can result in numbness and tingling, known as **paraesthesia**, or to anaesthesia of nearby skin due to nerve damage. Sometimes the end of a cut nerve at the margin of a wound develops a **neuroma**, a tender nodule of nerve fibres and cells which forms as the nerve tries to regenerate.

Swelling of a limb may follow lymph node excision. Although it is usually minor, it can occasionally be more significant, causing discomfort and limitation of function. Support with a compression stocking may then be necessary, with intermittent compression therapy in severe cases.

CHAPTER 9

Radiotherapy

> * A **radiologist** is a doctor trained to interpret X-rays and in the administration of dyes etc. which are used for some types of X-ray examination.
> * A **radiographer** is a technician who has undergone a three-year degree course and is qualified to operate X-ray machinery and to administer radiation treatment under the guidance of a doctor.
> * A **radiotherapist** (or **radiation oncologist**) is a doctor who specialises in the treatment of cancer using radiation. Most also administer other types of cancer treatment, such as chemotherapy.

WHEN IS RADIOTHERAPY APPROPRIATE?

Malignant melanomas are relatively resistant to radiation, and therefore surgery is the primary treatment for all patients with melanomas who are reasonably fit. The only real role for radiotherapy in the treatment of malignant melanomas is palliative (see p.96).

Radiotherapy can be used to treat most basal and squamous cell carcinomas although, as there is a small risk that irradiation can cause skin cancers to develop some 20 or 30 years later, it is usually a treatment reserved for older people.

When a suitably experienced plastic surgeon is not available, radiotherapy may be an alternative to surgery for the treatment of skin cancers at sites which are difficult to operate on. Examples include basal cell carcinomas on the lower eyelid, corner of the eye, lip, nose or ears. Radiotherapy may be the best option for very large squamous cell carcinomas (over about

5 cm), for those which have invaded cartilage or bone, for cancers which have recurred at the edge of an area of skin following surgical excision, and for multiple carcinomas. It is not appropriate for carcinomas in the middle of the upper eyelid as the resulting scar can scratch and damage the cornea of the eye.

There is sometimes a lack of consensus between surgeons and radiotherapists as to the relative merits of the two types of treatment, and you should not be afraid to ask your consultant about the anticipated cosmetic results and about other forms of treatment. Skin carcinomas are rarely life threatening, particularly basal cell carcinomas, and it is perfectly reasonable for you to be concerned about the affect treatment will have on your appearance. Doctors are generally far more sympathetic to this consideration than they were a few years ago.

WHAT IS RADIOTHERAPY?

Radiotherapy involves the use of ionising radiation (X-rays) to destroy malignant tissue. Although the X-rays damage the DNA in all cells in the targeted area, normal cells can usually repair themselves within a couple of hours, whereas the cancer cells cannot and, after repeated doses of radiation, are eventually relatively selectively destroyed. During treatment, the normal skin around the cancer is covered to protect it from radiation, and any reddening due to damage to it will only last for a couple of weeks.

Usually the radiation used to treat skin carcinomas penetrates only skin deep, leaving the deeper tissues of the body unharmed. Although surgery is often the treatment of choice for deeper-rooted skin cancers, radiotherapy can sometimes be delivered by a machine called a *linear accelerator* which uses electrons to control and vary the depth of penetration of the X-rays, to between about 2 and 7 cm.

TREATMENT SESSIONS

You may be sent an appointment for pre-treatment planning so that the doctor can decide how best to administer your radiotherapy.

Before your treatment starts, a total radiation dose is calculated and divided into several equal amounts to be given at each treatment session. Although different treatment centres may divide the total dose differently, the outcome is generally the same.

Radiation treatment of skin carcinomas is painless and is commonly given once a day for a week or more, sometimes three times a week, and occasionally eight or even ten times over a couple of weeks. A better cosmetic result can sometimes be obtained by dividing the total radiation dose into a larger number of fractions, and you should therefore tell the radiotherapist before your treatment begins if you are concerned about the cosmetic appearance. Each treatment session lasts only a few minutes.

The X-ray machine has a series of circular holes through which the radiation can be emitted, one of which may match the size and shape of your skin cancer. If not, the radiographer will select an appropriately shaped template. The template is made of lead, which blocks the passage of X-rays and protects the surrounding normal skin, and has a hole in it which is placed over the cancer itself.

Sometimes a plaster cast is made of the part of the body to be treated, from which an individual lead template can be constructed. However, where available, linear accelerators are now used to treat carcinomas of irregular shape or depth.

Very occasionally, low-dose radiation is administered by means of strips of radioactive metal (often irridium) embedded in a mould. The mould is put over the skin cancer and left in place for several hours, possibly for up to eight hours a day for five days, although treatment periods vary. This type of treatment involves a stay in hospital and allows a low dose of radiation to be delivered over a prolonged period, thus avoiding its absorption by underlying bone. However, the use of electrons is preferable when a linear accelerator is available.

During the pre-treatment planning or on your first visit for radiotherapy, a radiographer will explain the procedures to you. Do ask any questions, however trivial they may seem, and do not be afraid to ask for something to be explained again if you have not understood it. If you have any worries or questions as your treatment progresses, ask to talk to the radiographer again on a subsequent visit.

When you enter the treatment room for your first radiotherapy session, you will be asked to lie on a couch and the doctor will draw on your skin around the carcinoma with a felt-tip pen. If a template is being used, it will be taped to your skin, and the X-ray machine will be lowered until it almost touches the lesion. You will be told to keep very still while treatment is in progress.

Once the machine has been set up, all the medical staff will leave the treatment room to protect themselves against repeated exposure to radiation. A radiographer will watch you closely through a window or on a television monitor. If you are concerned or require any assistance, simply raise your hand and the process will be stopped immediately. There will also be an intercom system so the radiographer can hear and speak to you. The treatment only lasts a couple of minutes.

A scab may form over the lesion as the treatment sessions progress. If it is very thick, it may be removed by a doctor so that it does not affect the depth of tissue penetrated by the X-rays. You should not touch the scab and should definitely not pick it. Touching it can introduce infection, which may make it weep, redden and possibly become sore. Any infection should be reported to your family doctor or to the radiographer or doctor at the treatment centre so that antibiotics can be prescribed for you.

You may be given hydrocortisone cream to reduce any inflammation of the surrounding skin during the course of your treatment. Apart from anything which has been prescribed for you, do not put any type of cream, lotion or powder on your skin. Some creams which can be bought over the counter contain minute particles of metal which can deflect radiation onto the surrounding skin during radiotherapy.

Hostel wards Some hospitals have hostel wards, usually open from Monday to Friday, for use by people who would have to travel some distance each day for their treatment. The hostel wards provide people with a bed and meals during their stay, and although they are not staffed by nurses, there is always someone in charge of them. These wards are suitable for people who are able to look after themselves, and are therefore ideal for those undergoing daily radiotherapy treatment for skin carcinomas.

Do ask your doctor before your treatment starts about the availability of hostel ward beds if appropriate.

AFTER YOUR TREATMENT

Radiation to the scalp only induces hair loss in the area being treated. As the X-rays used to treat skin carcinomas only penetrate a short distance through the skin, they do not cause the sickness which can be associated with radiotherapy for cancers deeper in the body.

When your treatment is complete, a letter will be sent to your family doctor giving any relevant details and outlining any future care you may require. You will also be sent a date for a follow-up appointment.

Skin care

It is best to leave the skin open to the air to encourage healing, although a dressing may be used in the early stages to keep it clean or if there is a scab which causes you embarrassment. If you do have a dressing, arrangements will be made for a nurse to visit you at home to change it as necessary. The treated area should not be exposed to the sun for several weeks. In fact, irradiated skin will remain more sensitive to exposure to excessive sun, heat, cold, wind or injury.

The affected skin should be kept dry until it has healed. Even after your treatment has finished, the skin will be more sensitive than normal and you should therefore continue to avoid putting creams or lotions on it until healing is complete.

Once the skin has healed, it is likely to be paler and thinner than that around it, due to atrophy of the skin, and may be irregularly pigmented. There may be a scar, although how obvious this is will depend on the colour and texture of the surrounding skin. If you are distressed by its appearance, ask your family doctor to refer you for camouflage advice, sometimes available through the British Red Cross in Britain or from a clinic at a hospital. Alternatively, reconstructive surgery may be possible to replace the damaged skin.

Side-effects

The skin may redden during the last few days of treatment, a condition known as **erythema**. The colour is likely to deepen for about a week and then begin to fade. Once any scab falls off, the skin may be pigmented, but this also fades over weeks or months.

Later reactions to radiotherapy include a decrease or increase in pigmentation of the treated area (**hypopigmentation** or **hyperpigmentation**, respectively), wasting away (**atrophy**) of the skin, and occasionally multiple dilated blood vessels (**telangiectasia**). As already mentioned, the treatment itself may lead to the development of skin malignancies in the treated area in the long term.

Advanced skin cancer

RECURRENT DISEASE

The cure rate for skin cancers is very high, with the exception of some types of advanced melanomas and a rare group of squamous cell carcinomas which have metastasised. But all types of skin cancer may recur despite seemingly adequate treatment, and occasionally a new growth may arise locally from skin which has been damaged by ultraviolet radiation. Although the recurrence of cancer is always worrying, it may be treated by further surgery or by radiotherapy. If radiotherapy was the primary treatment and recurrence is very close to the primary area, it is not usually possible to repeat it as the surrounding normal cells are already likely to have had the maximum permissible dose of radiation. However, it is normally possible to repeat surgery if the cancer has recurred following surgical excision.

METASTATIC DISEASE

Any type of skin cancer can metastasise, particularly malignant melanoma, although it is very rare with basal cell carcinomas and only slightly less rare with squamous cell carcinomas. Most metastases develop when treatment has not been sought until the primary lesion is large or following recurrence of an aggressive skin cancer. The secondary lesions are normally treated surgically or with radiotherapy.

Metastatic disease can be local, regional or distant. *Local metastasis* occurs as the lesion extends horizontally and/or vertically. *Regional metastasis* results from the spread of malignant cells via the lymphatic vessels to the regional lymph nodes. *Distant metastasis* (usually of a malignant melanoma) can lead to the development of secondary lesions almost anywhere in the body, unlike most other types of cancer which tend to have a predictable pattern of spread. On the rare occasions that basal cell carcinomas do metastasise, spread is usually to the regional lymph nodes.

Malignant melanomas tend to spread first to the regional lymph nodes, and then to other skin tissue, the brain, lungs, intestines, liver, spleen or bone. Metastasis of malignant melanomas is often associated with a poor prognosis. In the overwhelming majority of cases of malignant melanoma in which metastasis occurs, it does so first within three years of treatment of the primary lesion. Follow-up is therefore important, and you will be examined every three or four months for the first three years, and probably yearly thereafter.

When metastases occur in the regional lymph nodes, aggressive therapy is usually advocated, and surgery is almost always the treatment of choice at the present time. With more advanced disease, treatment may cause more distress than is warranted by its outcome, and it is therefore often limited to that which is necessary to relieve symptoms (see Chapter 11). However, an enormous amount of research is currently underway into skin cancers, and the situation could change in this field in a relatively short space of time. Any of the more promising lines of research could soon show benefits in terms of the treatment of advanced disease.

ADJUVANT THERAPY

An adjuvant therapy is one which increases the efficacy of the primary treatment when used in combination with it. The primary treatment for skin cancer is often surgery although, as explained in Chapter 9, radiotherapy may be the preferred option in particular cases. Radiotherapy may also be used under some circumstances as an adjuvant, as may chemotherapy and immunotherapy. But in the case of skin cancer, these treatments are normally reserved for recurrent or advanced metastatic disease, or for lesions which appear to be localised but which have a poor prognosis.

Before starting a course of adjuvant radiotherapy, chemotherapy or immunotherapy, or a combination of any of them, you will see a consultant in **clinical** or **medical oncology**. The oncologist will examine you and look at the results of your operation and of any investigations which have been done. You may need to have further tests, such as a liver or bone scan, to determine whether the cancer has spread to other sites in the body. The oncologist will then discuss the proposed treatment plan with you. Do not be afraid to keep asking questions until you are sure you understand what your treatment involves and the effects it may have.

Radiotherapy

Radiotherapy may be used in combination with surgery when neither is likely to effect a cure alone. It may occasionally be given before surgery in an attempt to shrink a lesion and make excision easier. However, it does cause loss of blood vessels in the treated area, which makes flap repair (which is dependent on a good blood supply) less likely to be successful.

Adjuvant radiotherapy is more commonly used post-operatively following excision which has had to remain incomplete for fear of damaging an adjacent organ. It can also be used as a safeguard if it has only been possible to excise a small margin around an aggressive cancer. When given as an adjuvant, radiotherapy is administered in the same way as described in Chapter 9.

Chemotherapy

Chemotherapy involves the use of drugs which are able (reasonably selectively) to destroy, or prevent the growth of, cancer cells without permanently damaging normal cells. The drugs can sometimes be applied topically as a cream, given as tablets or injected locally or systemically. Unlike radiotherapy, which attacks cancer cells in the specific area at which the X-ray beam is directed, the drugs used in chemotherapy can kill cancer cells throughout the body. It is sometimes used before radiotherapy to reduce the size of a lesion which cannot be treated surgically.

When you are assessed by the oncologist, the most appropriate drug and the timing and duration of treatment will be decided upon. A blood sample will be taken to assess your blood count, and you will be given the drugs by injection into the back of your hand or forearm, or as a combination of injections and tablets. Adjuvant chemotherapy is usually given in an out-patients' clinic over a period of four to six months.

Basal cell carcinoma
Chemotherapy is not often needed to treat basal cell carcinomas as these respond well to surgery or radiotherapy. However, topical treatment is sometimes given for superficial or extensive multiple basal cell carcinomas. The most common agents are colcemid and 5-fluorouracil, both of which are applied as creams twice daily for a limited period of time. You will be given instructions about how and when to use them. They are both very effective, although colcemid can cause inflammation of the surrounding skin.

Squamous cell carcinoma
Topical chemotherapy is not very effective in the treatment of squamous cell carcinomas, but systemic treatment has shown some success, albeit short lived. Drugs such as methotrexate, cisplatin, bleomycin, doxorubicin and 5-fluorouracil can be used

alone or in various combinations. However, chemotherapy alone cannot cure squamous cell carcinoma, although treatment with 5-fluorouracil before radiotherapy may help sensitise the lesion to radiation.

Malignant melanoma

Chemotherapy may be used as an adjuvant treatment for localised malignant melanoma which has ulcerated or when there is regional metastasis only. It is more useful, however, as a palliative treatment to reduce the symptoms of widespread metastases which cannot be cured (see Chapter 11).

The most effective chemotherapeutic agent for malignant melanoma is a substance called DTIC (or dacarbazine) which causes partial regression in some cases when used as an adjuvant to surgery. It can be given, for example, as five daily injections over a period of four weeks or once every four weeks for a variable length of time, and is used in combination with other drugs which help to prevent the body becoming resistant to it. The injections take about five to ten minutes to administer. Alternatively, a drip may be set up to deliver an infusion of DTIC over a period of about an hour. As the drug is inactivated by light, the bag containing the infusion and the tube used to deliver it will be covered with black plastic.

A group of substances called the vinca alkaloids are sometimes also used in chemotherapy for malignant melanoma. Vincristine and vinblastine are obtained from the periwinkle plant; vindesine is a synthetic analogue. The vinca alkaloids are administered every week or every two to four weeks, and vindesine is sometimes used in combination with DTIC when aggressive treatment is required.

Side-effects

Different drugs have different side-effects, and the doctor and chemotherapy nurse will explain these to you before your treatment begins. It is particularly important when drugs are used for palliation in cases of incurable cancer that the possible side-effects are balanced against their likely affect on relieving symptoms. You should make sure that you understand the possibilities before your treatment starts.

The most common side-effects are nausea, vomiting, tiredness, and effects on the blood count. Some drugs cause extensive hair loss, whereas others cause little or none. The side-effects of DTIC can be distressing, and include nausea and vomiting for several hours after each injection. DTIC is extremely irritating to the skin if it accidentally comes into contact with it, so great care needs to be taken during its injection. The vinca alkaloids can cause nausea, malaise and occasionally hair loss, and sometimes severe constipation and degeneration of the central or peripheral nerves, known as **neuropathy**.

All side-effects will stop as soon as the chemotherapy comes to an end. Any hair which has been lost will grow back as thick as it was before, sometimes thicker. Wigs are available for both men and women who suffer hair loss, and arrangements can be made for you to be fitted for one at the local hospital or oncology centre.

Do discuss with the doctor or nurse any side-effects you experience as it may be possible for you to be given something to reduce the symptoms.

Regional chemotherapy

Also known as **isolated limb perfusion**, this treatment is sometimes used for recurrent malignant melanoma in a limb when surgery is inappropriate. It involves closing off the blood supply to and from the affected limb using a tourniquet applied under general anaesthesia.

A cannula (see p.56) is inserted into the major artery and vein carrying blood to and from the affected limb. The circulation of blood is taken outside the body and a cytotoxic drug is added to it. As the drug is unable to enter the blood going to other parts of the body, it may be given in high concentration without causing harmful toxic effects. The most commonly used agent is melphalan, sometimes in combination with actinomycin D.

This treatment seems to be effective for early melanoma with a poor prognosis and for slightly more advanced disease when used in combination with surgery. However, conclusive results of trials are not yet available.

Although regional chemotherapy cannot cure skin cancer, it does have quite good palliative results in many cases, but there is a significant incidence of local **lymphoedema** in the treated area. Lymphoedema is swelling caused by the collection of lymph which is unable to drain away. It can often be controlled by regular gentle exercise, massage and general skin care but, when severe, can be painful and debilitating.

Immunotherapy

Various substances may be used in an attempt to activate the body's own immune system in some cases of metastatic or recurrent malignant melanoma. Immunotherapy is never used to treat basal cell carcinomas, which normally respond to more established therapy. It was thought that as malignant melanoma gives rise to an immune response, it should respond to an anti-cancer treatment based on manipulation of the body's own immune system. But immunotherapy has so far proved to be of little value in the treatment of this type of cancer.

The injection of bacille Calmette Guerin (BCG) – commonly used as a vaccine against tuberculosis – into small recurrent melanomas can be effective in some cases, but apparently no more so than surgery or radiotherapy, and this agent is now rarely used.

The interferons (INFs) – proteins which occur naturally within the body and which act against a wide range of viruses – have sometimes been found to be effective in treating metastatic melanoma, particularly when used in combination with dacarbazine. Their side-effects include chills, nausea and vomiting, but are seldom severe. Evidence seems to suggest that, in some cases, interferon given after surgery can improve survival.

Interleukin 2 (IL2) is another naturally occurring substance which stimulates the production of the body's own disease-fighting cells (the T-lymphocytes) and which may be useful as an adjuvant or for palliation of advanced disease.

Tumour necrosis factor (TNF) is one of a group of proteins responsible for cell regulation within the body. It has been used in clinical trials for the treatment of malignant melanoma, but so far without any significant success.

FUTURE DEVELOPMENTS

With the realisation that cancer cells do not have the regulatory mechanisms of normal cells which control their growth and death, the emphasis is now shifting towards finding a treatment which damages cancer cells and leads them, in effect, to commit suicide. As the complex and subtle workings of cancer cells become better understood, more effective treatment should become available.

CHAPTER 11

Palliative care

W̲hen skin cancer is very advanced and cannot be cured, the use of chemotherapy, radiotherapy or immunotherapy may slow its growth or help relieve its symptoms. Radiotherapy, for example, may be useful in controlling ulceration, bleeding, infection and pain in an incurable skin cancer. This type of treatment, which may bring relief from symptoms and may even prevent the cancer from growing for many months or years, but which cannot cure it, is called palliation. Palliative care is not just for people who are about to die; it is long-term care that can continue for months or years.

There is now much that can be done to make living with incurable cancer a less frightening and stressful experience and to improve the quality of life for sufferers and their families. Care and support are available from hospices and specially trained nurses based in hospitals, cancer centres and the community.

In the UK, hospice-based care and the support of Macmillan nurses (see below) are free to all who need them, and are funded by charities or by the National Health Service.

HOSPICES

For those whose skin cancer has spread to other parts of their body to an extent which means it is not curable, hospice involvement may be suggested by their family doctor, consultant or a specialist cancer nurse. Many people are shocked at this suggestion as they imagine hospices to be places to go to die. But although some people choose to spend their last days in a hospice, their main role is to support cancer patients, and their families, and to help them remain well and to live as full and normal a life as possible for as long as possible – which in many cases means continuing support for years. Hospice staff work with family doctors to plan the best care for their patients.

Hospices have several aims:

* to help cancer patients live full and happy lives,
* to provide pain relief and to control any other symptoms of cancer which may arise,
* to counsel and support cancer patients and their families,
* to offer financial advice and information about grants and financial assistance which may be available,
* to provide education and courses on palliative care for nurses and doctors,
* to provide regular home visits to support and care for cancer patients and their families and enable people to be cared for in their own homes rather than in hospitals.

Some hospices also have in-patient facilities where people can go if they have symptoms which need to be brought under control, or simply to give their carers at home a week or two's respite. Many also have day-care facilities where cancer sufferers can spend the day involved in leisure activities such as painting, woodwork or making jewellery, and where they can have their hair done, be bathed if this is becoming difficult at home, talk to a doctor or social worker, or just sit and chat in a friendly and supportive environment.

Specialist nurses based within hospices or in the community work closely with family doctors – who remain in overall charge of their patients' care – as well as with community nurses and social workers. Their special skills and experience enable them to co-ordinate the care their patients receive and to make sure they have the emotional support and medical treatment they require.

Some people prefer not to be referred to a hospice, and some manage well alone. But many who do accept this help find their quality of life and ability to cope with their disease much improved.

MACMILLAN NURSES

The Cancer Relief Macmillan Fund (CRMF) was set up in the UK in 1911 to provide care and support for cancer patients. This national charity now helps to improve the quality of life for cancer patients and their families at home, in hospitals and in special cancer units.

The CRMF has trained over a thousand Macmillan nurses who work in the community and in hospitals around Britain. It continues to fund these specially trained nurses for up to three years in posts in hospitals, after which financial responsibility is taken over by the health authority.

A doctor or district nurse may suggest involving a Macmillan nurse to help care for someone with incurable skin cancer. Macmillan nurses play a similar role to that of hospice-based nurses, giving advice and emotional support to patients and their families, and working closely with other medical professionals to advise about pain relief and symptom control as necessary. They are also involved in the training of doctors and nurses to help them develop the special skills required for the care of cancer patients and, with hospice staff, have been largely responsible for the increased awareness of other health professionals to the particular care these patients need.

OTHER TREATMENT CENTRES

The effects of complementary or alternative therapies are difficult to assess, in part because they are often only resorted to by people for whom conventional medicine has no more to offer in terms of cure.

There are a few private centres in Britain which advocate special non-medical therapies to help people 'fight' or live with cancer. Your family doctor, consultant or a specialist nurse should be able to give you details of any such centres in your area, or you can contact one of the associations whose addresses are given in Appendix V. Alternative therapy centres are not funded by the NHS, but some have trust funds to help meet the costs for those who cannot afford them.

CHAPTER 12

Private care

In countries such as Britain where there is a state health service, there are various reasons why people choose to be treated privately. They may have private health insurance, or be covered by a private health scheme run by the company for which they work, or they may be able to pay for private care themselves. Whatever your situation, you will not find that the *standard* of medical care you receive in a private hospital is any different from that available on the National Health Service. But you may prefer the privacy of a private hospital; or you may find it convenient to be able to enter hospital for an operation more or less at the time of your choice. However, if you are being treated as an NHS patient and your doctor suspects you have skin cancer, arrangements will be made for you to see a specialist and to receive any necessary treatment with the minimum of delay.

If you have an operation in an NHS hospital, you may not see the consultant at all, being examined and treated by different doctors in the consultant's firm. At a private hospital, you will receive personal care from the consultant throughout your stay, whether you are having surgery, radiotherapy or chemotherapy. Although chemotherapy can be administered in a private hospital, it is rare for private hospitals in Britain to have their own, expensive, radiation equipment, and radiotherapy is therefore likely to be done at an NHS centre, by NHS staff under the supervision of your private consultant. You will probably be admitted to a private bed on an NHS ward if you require in-patient treatment. For some people, the fact that they will see their consultant at all follow-up appointments, and not different doctors in the consultant's firm, is an added advantage of private treatment.

The information given in other chapters in this book is equally relevant whichever system you choose. This chapter deals with the aspects of private health care which differ from those of the NHS.

PRIVATE HEALTH INSURANCE

If you work for a company which has a private health insurance scheme, your Company Secretary will be able to give you details, and should be able to tell you if the company insurance covers you for your treatment.

If you have your own private health insurance, the insurance company will be able to tell you exactly what is covered by your particular policy, if this is not clear from the literature you already have. It is always worth checking anyway, and asking for written confirmation. Do not be afraid to keep asking questions until you are certain you know exactly which costs you will be responsible for paying yourself. For example, does your insurance cover all follow-up appointments?

There are different levels of health insurance, and you need to read your policy carefully to make sure you know which costs are included. Most private hospitals have an administration officer who will check your policy for you if you are in any doubt. The staff at the hospital are likely to be very helpful and will try to sort out any problems and queries you have. But do read your policy carefully, and any information sent to you by the hospital, as unexpected charges, such as consultants' fees which may not be covered by your insurance policy, could add up to quite a lot of money.

With some types of private health insurance, you will need to ask your family doctor to fill in a form stating that your treatment is necessary and cannot be done in an NHS hospital within a certain time period due to long waiting lists. You will have to pay your doctor for this service, which will cost a few pounds. This money is not redeemable from your insurers.

FIXED PRICE CARE

If you think you may be able to pay to have private treatment, the Bookings Manager at a private hospital can give you an idea of the cost involved. Some private hospitals run a service known as Fixed Price Care: a price can be quoted to you before you enter hospital which covers your treatment and a variety of other hospitalisation costs. You should always ask to have the quotation in writing *before* you enter hospital, with a written note of everything it includes. At some hospitals, the fixed price will include accommodation, nursing, meals, drugs, dressings, operating theatre fees, X-rays etc.; at others only some of these are included. Once you have a written quotation, you should not have to worry about any hidden costs for which you had not accounted. However, the price quoted to you by the hospital may not include the fees of the consultant surgeon or anaesthetist, and you may have to ask your consultant for a note of these.

With Fixed Price Care, all the hospitalisation costs included by that particular hospital are covered should a complication arise which is directly related to your skin cancer or its treatment and which necessitates you staying longer in hospital, usually up to a maximum of 28 days. Again, consultants' fees may be extra. However, if you develop some problem while in hospital which is unrelated to the skin cancer, the price you have been quoted will not cover treatment to deal with this. At some hospitals, the quoted price will also include your treatment should you have to be re-admitted due to a complication related to your original treatment and arising within a limited period of time after your discharge.

The only extra charges you will have to pay to the hospital will probably include those for telephone calls, any alcohol you have with your meals, food provided for your visitors, personal laundry done by the hospital, hairdressing, and for any similar items such as you would have to pay for in a hotel. It is usually possible for a visitor to eat meals with you in your room, and for tea and snacks to be ordered for visitors during the day. (You will also have to pay these extra charges before you leave the hospital if you are being treated under private health insurance.)

It is important therefore that you ask in advance for *written confirmation* of the price you will have to pay for your stay in hospital and what is included in the quotation. If the hospital does not have a Fixed Price Care or similar system, make sure that all possible costs are listed.

ARRANGING AN OPERATION

Although the treatment you receive in a private hospital will be similar to that available at any NHS hospital, there are some basic differences between the two systems.

As with the NHS, you will have to be referred to see a consultant privately by your family doctor. Most doctors have contacts with particular consultants (and private hospitals) to whom they tend to refer patients. If there is a private hospital you particularly want to go to, or a consultant you have some reason to prefer, you can ask your family doctor to make an appointment for you.

After the visit to your doctor, you are unlikely to have to wait longer than a week or two before you see the consultant at an out-patient appointment. Your appointment may be at the private hospital where your operation is to be carried out, at an NHS hospital which has private wards, or at the consultant's private consulting rooms. Once the decision has been made to go ahead with an operation, you will probably be able to enter hospital at your convenience within another week or two.

You will receive confirmation of the date of your operation from the hospital's Bookings Manager. You will also probably be sent leaflets and any further relevant details of how to prepare for your admission to hospital. Do read these carefully, as knowing how a particular hospital organises things will help you to be prepared when you arrive for your operation. You will also be sent a *pre-admission form* to fill in and take with you when you are admitted.

If your operation is being paid for by insurance, you will be asked to take a completed insurance form with you when you are admitted to hospital. You should have been given some of these forms when you first took out your policy, but your insurance company will be able to supply the correct one if you have any problems. If you are covered by company insurance, the form will probably be filled in and given to you by your Company Secretary.

ADMISSION AND DISCHARGE

When you arrive at the hospital, the receptionist will contact the admissions department, and a ward receptionist will come to collect you. If you are paying for your stay in hospital yourself, you will probably be asked to pay your bill in advance at this stage, if you have not already done so. Otherwise, you will be asked for your completed insurance form. The ward receptionist will take you to your room – probably a single or double room – and show you the facilities available there. You are likely to have a private bathroom, a television, and a telephone by your bed. The ward receptionist will explain hospital procedures to you, and will leave you to settle in.

A member of the nursing staff will then come to make a note of your medical details, in much the same way as described in

Chapter 4. The main difference you are likely to notice if you have been treated in an NHS hospital before, is that this time there is much less waiting for all the routine hospital procedures to be dealt with. The nurse to patient ratio is higher in private hospitals and so someone is usually available to deal with the pre-operative procedures quite quickly.

Your consultant will take charge of your medical care throughout your stay, will visit you before the operation, perform the operation (with the assistance of the anaesthetist and the operating staff), and visit you again when you are back in your own room. Trainees – whether doctors or nurses – do not work in private hospitals. The consultants are responsible for their own patients and supervise their care themselves. Most private hospitals now have resident medical officers – fully qualified, registered doctors who are available 24 hours a day to deal with any emergencies which may arise.

If you are having a general anaesthetic, when the time for your operation approaches a porter and nurse will take you from your room to the anaesthetic room. In many private hospitals, you will not be moved from your bed onto a trolley until you have been anaesthetised; the bed itself will be wheeled from your room. Similarly, you will be transferred back from the trolley to your own bed in the recovery room while you are still asleep. You therefore go to sleep and wake up in your own hospital bed.

If you are having a local anaesthetic, you may be taken to the operating theatre in a wheelchair.

Your operation will be performed in the same way as described in Chapter 6, and when you are fully awake, you will be taken back to your room to rest.

When you are ready to be discharged from hospital, the ward receptionist will ask you to pay any outstanding charges not covered by the hospitalisation charge. You will be given any medical items you may need from the hospital pharmacy.

SUMMARY

The main aim of the staff of any private hospital is the same as that in an NHS hospital – to make your stay as pleasant and as comfortable as possible. Because the staffing ratio is higher in private hospitals, more emphasis can be placed on privacy and comfort.

The consultant surgeons and anaesthetists almost always work in NHS hospitals as well as in a private hospital, so you will receive the same expertise and skill under both systems. However, in an NHS hospital you may not actually be operated on by the consultant surgeon who heads the surgical team and, indeed, you may not see the consultant at all during your stay.

Private hospitals arrange their operating lists differently from NHS hospitals. The NHS hospitals have 'sessional bookings' for their operating theatres, which means that a particular day is set aside at regular intervals for a specialist in one type of surgery to perform operations. In private hospitals, the consultants can book the use of an operating theatre (and the assistance of the staff who work in it) on more or less any day, at any time that suits them. Therefore, your operation should be able to take place privately at a time that is convenient to you and your consultant.

It is also possible, even if you are already on an NHS waiting list, to tell your family doctor or consultant at any time that you would like to change to private care. If the consultant you have already seen under the NHS does not have a private practice, you can ask to be put in touch with a consultant who *can* see you privately.

There are several reasons why, if they can, some people choose to have their operations done privately, either paid for by private health insurance or from their own pockets. Some find it more convenient to be able to have a say in when their operation is to take place. Some simply prefer the smaller, more intimate setting they are likely to find in a private hospital. As private hospitals rarely deal with accidents and emergency treatment (the operations carried out in them normally being planned at least a day or two in advance), they do not have the bustle of an NHS hospital which has to deal with emergency admissions as well as the routine admissions for non-emergency operations.

Although the NHS, under which the majority of people are treated in Britain, naturally has longer waiting lists, the treatment of skin cancer will always be carried out with the minimum of delay.

Questions and answers

1. *I have always had several moles on my back, but recently noticed a new one. It doesn't itch or irritate in any way, so is it safe to assume that it is harmless?*

If your new mole is identical to those already present, it is unlikely to be a cause for concern. However, a new mole which is different from existing ones can indicate malignancy and, as early treatment can improve the outcome for all types of skin cancer, it should be shown to your doctor.

2. *I recently saw a consultant because I have a small patch of brownish skin on my arm which has grown bigger over the last few months. The consultant says it is nothing to worry about, but I am anxious about it and would like it to be removed. Can I go back to the consultant and ask to have it cut away?*

If your consultant had *any* doubts about your skin lesion, he or she would have taken some action. However, your concerns should be viewed sympathetically, and you could ask your doctor or the consultant to explain what the lesion is and why no treatment is necessary. It may be possible for it to be removed to put your mind at rest, although you should bear in mind that the resulting scar may be more obvious than the lesion itself. Do discuss your worries with your doctor, who may make another appointment for you to see the consultant. But do be reassured if both are satisfied that all is well.

3. I am 50 years old and have a small basal cell carcinoma on my face which a dermatologist has suggested should be treated with radiotherapy. I would prefer to have it surgically removed as I am concerned about the use of radiation. Is my preference likely to be taken into account?

Your preference should always be taken into account. You may want to ask to be referred to a radiotherapist or clinical oncologist to find out more about radiotherapy, although your dermatologist should be able to explain the options to you. Do ask to see the dermatologist again, or another consultant, to discuss your concerns and the treatment options. Theoretically, surgery should be the treatment of choice for someone of your age, but if there is some reason why radiotherapy is more appropriate in your case, this should be explained to you. Do not be embarrassed to keep asking questions until you are satisfied that you understand what is being suggested and why.

4. Last summer, my 5-year-old son was quite badly sunburnt while on holiday. He has blond hair and fair skin, and I am worried about whether this incident may lead to his getting skin cancer in later life. What are the chances of this happening, and is there anything I can now do to lessen the risk?

It is impossible to say what the chances are of your son developing skin cancer in later life after a single episode of sunburn. There are other factors involved, and no simple relationship exists between skin cancer and sun exposure alone. However, to reduce any future risk, always make sure your son's skin is protected from sun exposure by loose clothing and that any exposed areas of skin are covered with a high factor sunscreen preparation, even when there is little direct sun. Try to keep him out of the sun when it is at its strongest, between 10 a.m. and 2 p.m., and make sure he wears a wide-brimmed sun hat and, whenever possible, proper sunglasses in strong sunlight.

5. I have quite a pale skin and look forward to getting brown each summer. Should I avoid the sun in future in case I get skin cancer?

Accepting that pale skin is attractive is the most significant step you can take towards avoiding skin cancer. Any sun exposure is damaging, especially around midday when the level of ultraviolet radiation is highest. If you really *must* get a tan, avoiding burning your skin may reduce the risk, although it will not remove it altogether.

6. I am going to Turkey on holiday in a few months. Is it best to tan my skin using a sunbed before I go so that I do not get sunburn on holiday?

Although at one time sunbeds were considered to be safer than the sun itself, this point of view is not now accepted. Sunbeds do utilise a type of ultraviolet light which damages the skin, and are therefore best avoided. Some evidence suggests that exposure to natural ultraviolet radiation after using a sunbed is more damaging than the sunlight alone. Although tanning gradually while on holiday is better than burning the skin by any method, it still results in long-term damage and the risk of skin cancer.

7. I had a malignant melanoma removed from my back a couple of years ago. Until then I used to spend a lot of time in the sun with my shirt off each summer, and did not use sun protection as a child when I lived by the sea. Although I am now careful to keep covered up in the sun, what are the chances that I will get another melanoma in the future?

It is very difficult to quantify your chances of getting another melanoma, but they may be as much as seven to ten times higher than for someone who has not had a previous skin cancer. However, the risk can be reduced – although not eliminated – by avoiding unnecessary exposure to the sun in future.

Continued vigilance is important, and you should examine your skin for new or altered lesions at regular intervals and consult your family doctor if you are concerned.

8. I am due to start a course of radiotherapy to treat a squamous cell carcinoma. Will the treatment make me feel sick or will I be able to return to work after each session?

Radiotherapy, when used for shallow-rooted skin cancers, does not cause sickness as the X-rays do not penetrate more than skin deep. There should be no reason why you cannot return to work after each treatment session, although you may feel quite tired during and possibly for a while after your treatment. Do discuss this with the radiotherapist if you are concerned. If possible, it may be sensible to have a contingency plan which allows you to work part time should you find the need to rest after each treatment session.

9. My father has to have a series of radiotherapy sessions on alternate days for a couple of weeks. He is elderly and it will be quite difficult for him to get to the hospital each time. Would it be possible for him to have one large dose of radiotherapy to get it all done with on one day?

As surgery has the advantage of being a one-off treatment, your father should perhaps discuss with his doctor whether it would be suitable in his case.

Radiotherapy is usually given in a series of small doses to avoid causing unnecessary damage to the normal skin cells. Normal cells are able to repair themselves to some extent after each session, whereas the malignant cells are gradually killed off. Therefore one large dose of radiation is not feasible. If there is some reason why your father should have radiotherapy rather than surgery, do ask at the radiotherapy centre if there is a hostel ward where he can stay each night during the week while his treatment continues. If he does stay in a hostel ward, he will be able to come and go as he likes but will be provided with meals and a bed at night so that he does not have to travel to and from the radiotherapy centre each day.

10. My family doctor says the small lump on my chest is nothing to worry about, but I am still concerned. I would like to see a specialist to make sure she is right, but do not want to offend her by asking her to arrange an appointment. Is there any other way I could see a consultant?

Your doctor may be confident that your lump is benign as she may have considerable experience of skin lesions. However, she should understand your anxiety and your desire to seek specialist confirmation of her diagnosis. Perhaps you could ask her about her level of experience, or write to her if you are embarrassed at the prospect of raising the matter face to face. Even if you see a consultant privately, your family doctor should be informed and you should ask her for a referral. However, under the circumstances you describe, most consultants would be willing to see you privately without prior referral, although they would have to inform your doctor after the event.

11. My wife has recently been diagnosed as having a malignant melanoma. Although I understood that this is a type a cancer, the doctor was very reassuring and says there is no cause for concern. He is making an appointment for her to see a plastic surgeon. Is the condition life threatening, and is he keeping the bad news from us?

Malignant melanoma *is* a type of skin cancer which, in its later stages of development, can spread both locally and to other parts of the body. When spread occurs, the outcome can be more serious and, in some cases, life threatening. However, if your doctor says there is no cause for concern, it is likely that the melanoma has been detected at an early stage when treatment is usually successful and the prognosis is good. Your wife may need to be examined at regular intervals, possibly for the next five years, to look for any signs of spread of the cancer. Do discuss your worries with the plastic surgeon, who should give you as honest a prognosis as possible, particularly if you ask clear, straightforward questions.

12. A small mark on my arm has been diagnosed as a basal cell carcinoma. Is this likely to spread to other parts of my body?

Basal cell carcinomas very rarely spread, but do ask the consultant for an opinion about your specific case.

13. My elderly mother has a malignant melanoma which has apparently spread quite extensively. She says she does not want treatment, except any which is absolutely necessary to make her feel better. I think she should try to fight the disease. Can I insist to her doctor that she does?

Although it must be very distressing for you to have to come to terms with what you may see as your mother's acceptance of defeat by her cancer, do try to support her in her decision. If she and her doctor realise there is very little chance of her recovering from very advanced cancer, it would cause her unnecessary pain and distress to undergo aggressive treatments to no avail. Once malignant melanoma is widespread, there really is very little likelihood of cure, although much can be done to relieve her symptoms. However, there is a great deal of support available for both your mother and yourself to help you to cope. Your doctor will be able to give you details of support groups, Macmillan nurses and hospice care. Your mother could gain a good deal from the facilities available at a hospice, which she can use as a day centre for support and company as well as for medical assistance. There are several support networks for the families of people with cancer, and you may find it helpful to talk to people in a similar situation as yourself. Do take advantage of all the assistance available to help you to understand and support your mother's decision, and to deal with the problems and worries which may arise.

Case histories

The case histories which follow are not intended to make any specific point. They have been chosen at random as examples of the experiences of different men and women who have had treatment for skin cancer.

CASE 1

James is 78. He has had warts on his back for many years, and a couple of years ago developed several small, pink, flat lesions on his face, which were diagnosed as keratoses and largely responded to treatment with an ointment. However, when a more pronounced pink lesion developed on his right cheek, he was referred by his family doctor to a dermatologist who excised it. Histological examination proved it to be a malignant melanoma (lentigo maligna). After a while, the lesion returned and James was referred to a plastic surgeon. The new melanoma was relatively superficial and he was admitted to hospital shortly afterwards for day-case surgery. The lesion was excised under a local anaesthetic and the wound was closed with several small stitches. He was in hospital for about an hour and a half. The stitches were removed by the practice nurse at his doctor's surgery about a week later.

James was in the Middle East during the Second World War.

CASE 2

John is 61. About a year ago, his wife noticed a mole, about 2 cm in diameter, on the hairline near his temple. His family doctor suggested it should be removed by another local doctor with surgical facilities. But John did not feel confident about this suggestion, and instead went privately to a dermatologist who removed the mole under a local anaesthetic. Histological examination proved it to have been a malignant melanoma.

Six months later, a lump developed near John's ear, and he then saw an NHS dermatologist who referred him to a plastic surgeon. Shortly afterwards, he was admitted to hospital and the lump and the lymph nodes in his neck were excised under a general anaesthetic. Histology confirmed the presence of a metastatic melanoma in a lymph node.

John was in hospital for two weeks, which was rather longer than anticipated as fluid continued to drain from his tissues for longer than normal and the drain had to be left in place until the amount of fluid reduced. Although his shoulder was stiff after his operation, he did not experience any pain.

Some of the stitches were removed from the wound near his ear and in his neck about ten days after his operation, but as healing was incomplete, some were left in a little longer.

A few months later, one of John's knees became sore and during a follow-up appointment the surgeon noticed several small black spots on it. These were excised, but proved to be benign. John continues to return for a check-up every three months.

John spent most of his life in southern Africa, returning to live in England in 1985.

CASE 3

Martha is 83. About six years ago her family doctor removed a flat lesion near her ear by freezing it. A couple of years later, a basal cell carcinoma was excised from her cheek and shortly afterwards a brownish pink, raised lesion developed on her eyebrow. It did not cause her any concern at first, but when it grew and began to weep and form a crusty surface, she went to see her family doctor. A couple of weeks later a consultant took a biopsy, and within three weeks Martha entered hospital for day-case surgery. The lesion, which was another basal cell carcinoma, was excised under a local anaesthetic. Martha is due to return for a check-up in three months time.

Martha's father, who lived until he was 94, had a couple of basal cell carcinomas removed during his lifetime.

CASE 4

Susan is 28. She has always had several moles, but while on holiday recently a friend pointed out that one on her shoulder had grown larger, changed shape and darkened in colour. Susan went to her family doctor, who referred her to a plastic surgeon at a local hospital. The surgeon excised the mole immediately, using a local anaesthetic, and Susan was told that she would hear the results of a histological examination within a couple of weeks. When she had not heard anything two weeks later, she rang her family doctor, who contacted the hospital on her behalf. Susan's doctor then visited her at home to tell her that the lesion had proved to be a skin cancer – a superficial spreading malignant melanoma. Susan was very upset by the diagnosis as she thought that any type of cancer would spread throughout her body, but she was reassured by her doctor's explanations.

She returned to hospital a month later for the excision of a wider margin of skin. She found the second operation more distressing than the first: the local anaesthetic took longer to act and the surgeon needed to use additional anaesthetic before her shoulder was properly anaesthetised. An additional centimetre of tissue was excised all around the scar and the wound was closed with stitches.

Although the wound started to heal well, one end became sore after a couple of weeks and Susan returned to the hospital clinic. Some of the dissolvable stitches had caused a reaction and were being rejected by her body. Adhesive strips were put over the wound to keep it closed while it healed.

Four weeks after her operation, Susan was still having to be careful to avoid lifting and strenuous exercise which would put pressure on the wound. She will continue to be seen at intervals for the next few years.

Susan lived and worked in Cairo for three years in her early twenties.

CASE 5

Francis is 64 and is a diabetic with congestive heart failure and swollen legs. He had a wart-like growth on his right calf for 20 years or more, the top of which had been knocked off on two or three occasions. Each time, the lesion grew noticeably. On the last occasion, he took the severed section of tissue with him to show his family doctor, who sent it for histological examination. The doctor bandaged Francis' leg to protect the remains of the wart, which gradually healed. The laboratory report identified the lesion as a 'wart-like fungus'. However, the area of affected skin enlarged and became dry and itchy, and Francis was referred to a plastic surgeon.

When Francis was admitted to hospital to have the growth excised, a new, smaller lesion was found nearby. He was given a general anaesthetic and skin was taken from his left thigh to repair the two areas. Unfortunately, the skin around the grafts became inflamed and the bandages had to be removed. Although the larger skin graft gradually 'took', the smaller one did not, and the area was regrafted by a nurse on the ward using more of the skin which had been taken from Francis' thigh at the time of his operation. Histology showed both lesions to be squamous cell carcinomas.

Apart from a brief walk down the ward a couple of days after his operation, Francis was confined to bed with his leg raised for ten days. He was in hospital for 15 days, by which time both grafts had taken satisfactorily. He was able to manage quite well alone once at home, and was careful to take only short walks and to rest with his leg raised as much as possible.

A month or so after his operation, Francis still had a protective bandage over the grafts on his leg but was free from pain. In fact, the donor site had been the only real cause of any pain associated with his operation.

Medical terms

Abscess   A collection of pus secondary to localised infection.

Actinic keratosis/Solar keratosis/Sun wart   A scaly lesion which may be pink or brown. It is caused by excessive exposure to the sun and can transform into a squamous cell carcinoma.

Adjuvant therapy   A treatment used in combination with another, primary, treatment to enhance its efficacy.

Allergy   An abnormal reaction to a substance. An allergic reaction can be mild, causing an itchy rash, or severe, leading to fainting, vomiting, loss of consciousness or death.

Anaesthesia   The absence of sensation.

Anaesthetic   A drug which causes loss of sensation in part or all of the body.

Anaesthetist   A doctor trained in the administration of anaesthetics.

Analgesic   A drug which blocks the sensation of pain; a painkiller.

Antibiotic   A substance which kills bacteria or prevents them replicating.

Anti-embolism stockings   Stockings sometimes worn during an operation and during any period of immobilisation post-operatively. The stockings assist the circulation of blood in the legs and help to prevent blood clots forming.

Anti-emetic   A drug which helps to reduce feelings of sickness.

Atrophy   Wasting away due to lack of nourishment or use.

'Back slab'   Usually a plaster of Paris cast which is put around the back of a limb and may be held in place with bandages. It is sometimes used after a skin graft to support the leg and prevent the foot from drooping.

Basal cell   A cell in the basement layer of the epidermis of the skin.

Basal cell papilloma   *See* Seborrhoeic keratosis.

Basi-squamous   A colloquial name for a skin carcinoma which has characteristics of both a basal and a squamous cell carcinoma. It tends to be more aggressive, more likely to recur, and more likely to spread than either of the derivative forms.

Benign   Non-malignant. A benign disease or condition is likely to respond to appropriate treatment. A benign lesion will remain localised at its site of development and will have no harmful effect other than possibly to interfere with the function of adjacent organs as it grows.

Biopsy   The surgical removal of a piece of tissue from a living body for examination under a microscope to assist or confirm a diagnosis.

Bowen's disease   A lesion of the epidermis which is an early, non-invasive form of a squamous cell carcinoma.

Breslow's measurement   A method of determining the stage of development of a malignant melanoma based on its depth of invasion, measured in millimetres from the basal layer of the epidermis. The melanoma is classified as thin, intermediate or thick, the prognosis worsening progressively with each successive stage.

Cancer   A malignant growth resulting from the uncontrolled multiplication of cells which fail to die naturally. If left untreated, the cancer cells may invade nearby areas of the body and eventually spread to distant sites.

Cannula   A very fine tube or needle. Fluids can be introduced into or removed from the body through an intravenous cannula which has been inserted into a vein, usually in the back of the hand, and anaesthetic drugs are administered through it during an operation. Cannulas are usually made of plastic, but used to be metal or glass.

Carcinogen   A substance which causes cancer.

Carcinoma   A cancer in epithelial tissue which may spread locally and to distant sites in the body. Carcinomas are always malignant, but their severity and tendency to spread can vary.

Cataract   Opacity of the normally transparent lens of the eye which causes blurring of vision.

Chemotherapy   Treatment with drugs.

Cicatricial basal cell carcinoma   A malignant lesion with a diffuse margin and a central scar-like appearance. It tends not to increase in thickness, but growth occurs at the periphery and spread across the skin can be extensive.

Clark's level   A method of staging malignant melanomas to determine their level of development, from level 1 (in situ) to level 5 (the most invasive stage).

Co-carcinogen   A substance which acts with another to cause cancer.

Complication   A condition which occurs as the result of another disease or condition. It may also be an unwanted side-effect of treatment.

Congenital   Present from birth.

Connective tissue   Fibrous tissue which connects and supports organs within the body.

Consent form   A form which patients must sign before surgery to confirm that they understand what is involved in their oper-ation and give their consent for it to take place. Signing the form also gives consent for the use of anaesthetic drugs and any other procedures which doctors feel to be necessary during surgery.

Consultant   An experienced and fully trained doctor who specialises in a particular type of medicine.

Curettage   A procedure involving the use of a spoon-shaped scraping instrument (a curette) to remove tissue.

Curette   A spoon-shaped surgical instrument used for scraping.

Cyst   A fluid-filled swelling.

Cytological examination   The examination of cells under a microscope for the purposes of diagnosis.

Day-case surgery   Surgery for which a patient is in hospital for one day only, with no overnight stay.

Deep vein thrombosis (DVT)   A blood clot in a deep vein, often in the lower leg or pelvis.

Dermatofibroma/Sclerosing angioma   A benign, fibrous, pink lesion which may develop at the site of an insect bite.

Dermatologist   A physician who specialises in the treatment of skin diseases.

Dermis   The layer of skin below the epidermis.

Diagnosis   The identification of a disease based on its symptoms and signs.

Diathermy   A method of generating heat by means of a high-frequency electric current. It is used in surgery to destroy diseased tissue or to stop bleeding from damaged blood vessels.

Direct closure   The drawing together of the edges of a wound with stitches.

Discharge letter   A letter given to a patient leaving hospital (or sent directly from the hospital) to deliver to their family doctor. It gives details of treatment and any necessary follow-up.

Distant metastasis   Spread of malignant cells via the blood or lymphatic vessels to sites which are distant from the primary cancer.

Donor site   The site from which skin is removed to be transferred elsewhere.

Drain   Often a tube, which may be attached to a bag or bottle, which is inserted into a wound to drain away excess blood and fluid.

Drip   A tube used to administer fluid to replace that lost from the body after an operation or injury. One end is inserted into a vein in an arm and the other end is attached to a bottle or bag containing a specially balanced saline or sugar solution.

Dysplastic naevus   An abnormally shaped, benign mole with malignant potential.

Electrocardiogram (ECG)   The activity of the heart recorded as a series of electrical wave patterns.

Electromagnetic radiation   Any energy source emitted in wave form, including visible light, radio waves, gamma waves etc.

Embolus (plural: **emboli**)   A piece of a blood clot (or air bubble) which has broken away and can pass through the blood vessels. If it lodges in a vital organ, such as the lung, it can have fatal consequences.

Epicryosurgery   Destruction of the cells of a skin lesion by freezing. The frozen tip of an instrument called a **cryoprobe** is inserted into the lesion to freeze the cells, which are then allowed to thaw. The procedure is repeated, and over the ensuing weeks the damaged tissue dies and falls away.

Epicryotherapy   Freezing of the *surface* of the skin which may be done, for example, to destroy the cells of actinic keratoses and some superficial basal cell carcinomas.

Epidermis   The outer cellular layer of the skin.

Epidural anaesthetic   An anaesthetic drug which is injected into the space around the nerves in the back. It causes numbness in the legs and groin which lasts for three to five hours. Epidurals are used for pain relief and/or to produce loss of sensation during surgery to the legs or lower body.

Erythema   Redness due to increased blood flow.

Excision   Removal by cutting.

Excision biopsy   The surgical removal of an entire lesion from a living body.

Familial atypical naevus syndrome   A hereditary condition with an increased risk of melanoma, typified by multiple dysplastic naevi.

Fixed Price Care   The system used by some private hospitals whereby a fixed price is quoted for a particular type of operation and some of the hospitalisation costs associated with it.

Free skin flap/Microvascular flap   A flap of skin with some blood vessels attached which is removed from a donor site and used to repair or replace skin at another (recipient) site. The blood vessels are re-attached to those at the recipient site by means of microsurgical techniques, enabling the blood supply to the skin flap to be established immediately.

Full-thickness skin graft   A graft made from a segment of skin comprising epidermis and the entire depth of the dermis, and sometimes fat or cartilage. The donor skin is often taken from the neck or in front of or behind the ear.

General anaesthetic   A drug which induces loss of consciousness and abolishes the sensation of pain in all parts of the body.

Genetic predisposition   The likelihood of a person developing a particular disease which is dependent on their genetic make-up. Some diseases occur in members of the same family who share common genes.

Giant congenital hairy naevus   A large, hairy mole (greater than 20 square centimetres in area) which is present from birth.

Gorlin's syndrome   An inherited condition involving various skin disorders and abnormalities of the nervous and skeletal systems.

Graft   A piece of tissue removed from one site and placed at another to repair a defect resulting from an operation, accident or disease.

Haemangioma   A benign vascular lesion.

Haematoma   A blood-filled swelling. A haematoma can form in a wound after an operation if blood continues to leak from a blood vessel. If the blood spreads in the tissues, it appears as a bruise.

Heparin   A substance which occurs naturally in the body and which helps to prevent the blood clotting. It may be given by injection before and after surgery to people who are at particular risk of developing blood clots, for example during long periods of immobilisation.

Hereditary condition   A disease or condition transmitted from one generation to another; an inherited condition.

Histological examination   The microscopic examination of a sample of tissue which has been taken from the body by biopsy.

Hostel ward   A hospital ward set aside for people who do not need medical care but who are unable to go home immediately after an operation or between treatment sessions. Food and a bed are provided, but although there is always someone in charge of the ward, it does not have a full medical staff.

Human papilloma virus   The virus which causes viral warts.

Hydrocortisone   A steroid which occurs naturally in the body and which reduces inflammation. Synthetic hydrocortisone is used to treat various inflammatory and allergic conditions.

Hyperpigmentation   Excess pigment in a tissue.

Hypertrophy   Enlargement of a tissue or organ due to an increase in the number or size of its cells.

Hypopigmentation   Loss of pigment.

Immunological treatment/Immunotherapy   Treatment (usually involving the use of drugs) which activates the body's own immune mechanisms to fight disease.

Incidence   The rate of occurrence of new cases of, for example, a disease in a defined population in a specified period of time.

Incision   A cut or wound made by a sharp instrument, such as during an operation.

Incision biopsy   The surgical removal of part of a lesion from a living body.

Induction agent   A drug used in anaesthesia to bring on loss of consciousness.

Inhalational anaesthetic   An anaesthetic given as a mixture of gases which is inhaled, usually to maintain anaesthesia.

In-situ   Not invading outside its site of origin.

In-situ melanoma A malignant melanoma at an early stage of development which is confined within the epidermis and has not begun to invade the dermis.

Interferon A protein produced by the body in response, for example, to a virus, which inhibits its development. Interferon is used in immunotherapy in an attempt to stimulate the immune system.

Interleukin A substance produced by the body to stimulate the disease-fighting T-lymphocytes. It is sometimes used as an adjuvant or for palliation for advanced malignant melanoma.

Intra-epidermal carcinoma An in-situ squamous cell carcinoma which develops within the epidermis of the skin as a pink, scaly lesion. It expands slowly and may eventually become invasive.

Intra-operative Occurring during an operation.

Intravenous anaesthetic A general anaesthetic drug which is injected into a vein via a cannula, usually in the back of the hand.

Invasion The infiltration of malignant cells into adjacent normal tissue.

Invasive melanoma A stage in the development of a malignant melanoma during which it grows downwards into the dermis of the skin.

Isolated limb perfusion/Regional chemotherapy A treatment sometimes used for recurrent malignant melanoma in a limb. The blood supply to and from the limb is closed off using a tourniquet, and a cannula is inserted into the major artery and vein. The circulation is thus taken outside the limb so that a cytotoxic drug can be introduced into it without entering the general circulation of the body.

Kaposi's sarcoma A slowly developing malignant lesion which often occurs on the legs or feet. One type is common in elderly men of Mediterranean or Jewish descent; another is endemic in central Africa; and another can arise following immunosuppression therapy for organ transplantation. A more aggressive type is associated with AIDS and HIV infection.

Keloid   An abnormal scarring reaction characterised by continued growth of scar tissue once a wound has healed. It can occur spontaneously for reasons which are not understood.

Keratinocyte   A cell within the epidermis of the skin which takes up melanin from the melanocytes and transports it through the epidermis. Keratinocytes divide as they migrate through the epidermis, and eventually form a tough layer of dead cells on the skin's surface which are continuously rubbed off and replaced.

Keratoacanthoma   A benign, rapidly growing skin lesion, commonly on sun-exposed parts of the body, which may resemble a squamous cell carcinoma but which heals spontaneously after a few months.

Lentigo maligna   A type of malignant melanoma which often develops on the faces of elderly people or on other parts of the body regularly exposed to the sun. It is a slow-growing lesion which is flat in its early stages, with an irregular outline and brownish pigmentation. It may thicken and develop nodules at a late stage.

Lesion   Any abnormality such as an injury, infection or tumour.

Linear accelerator   A machine which emits a special type of radiation able to penetrate through the skin to a depth of about 2 cm. It may be used in radiotherapy to treat some deep-rooted skin cancers.

Local anaesthetic   An anaesthetic which numbs the area of the body around which it is injected.

Local injection   An injection of a substance which remains confined to one area and is not distributed throughout the body.

Local metastasis   Spread of malignant cells confined to the area immediately around the primary site.

Lymph   A pale-coloured fluid which flows within the lymphatic vessels of the body and is eventually returned to the blood. It contains disease-fighting cells, the lymphocytes.

Lymph node   A nodule through which lymph flows and is filtered and which acts as a home for the lymphocytes.

Lymphocyte   A type of white blood cell involved in fighting disease in the body.

Lymphoedema   A condition in which the lymphatic drainage of part of the body is impaired, causing swelling, tightness of the skin and pain as the lymph collects.

Lymphoma   A solid cancer of the lymphoid tissue, such as Hodgkin's disease or mycosis fungoides.

Maintenance agent   A drug used during an operation to maintain the state of general anaesthesia.

Malignant   Used to describe a lesion which is likely to spread locally and to distant parts of the body – a cancer.

Malpighian layer   A basal layer of the epidermis of the skin.

Melanin   A dark-coloured pigment present in the skin, hair etc.

Melanocyte   A cell which produces melanin.

Melanocytic naevus   A mole composed of pigment-containing cells (melanocytes).

Melanoma   A skin cancer caused by malignant melanocytes which may be pigmented or unpigmented.

Metastasis (noun; plural **metastases**)   A secondary cancer at a site distant from the original (primary) cancer.

Metastasis (verb)   The spread of cancerous cells through the blood or lymphatic vessels from the site of the original cancer.

Metastasise   To spread to a distant part.

Metastatic disease   Advanced cancer due to the spread of malignant cells from the primary lesion.

Microsurgery   Surgery involving the use of very small, fine instruments and a microscope.

Microvascular flap   *See* Free skin flap.

Mohs chemosurgery   A procedure involving the progressive removal of a circular piece of tissue from a skin cancer and its examination under a microscope. The procedure is repeated at progressively deeper levels until no further malignant cells can be detected.

Mole   A generic name for a fleshy skin growth which is usually pigmented but which can be white, hairy or warty.

Naevus   A mole or similar skin abnormality.

National Health Service (NHS)   The system of medical care, set up in Britain in 1948, under which medical treatment is mostly funded by taxation.

Nausea   A feeling of sickness.

Neoplasm   Any new formation of tissue; a tumour.

Nerve block   An anaesthetic which is injected near a particular nerve to cause loss of sensation in the area supplied by that nerve.

Neuroma   A tumour of nerve cells and nerve fibres.

Neuropathy   A condition involving the destruction or degeneration of the tissue of the central or peripheral nerves, caused by drugs or metabolic or vascular disturbance.

Nil by mouth   A term used to mean that no food or drink should be swallowed in the hours before an operation.

Nodule   A small swelling of cells.

Obesity   An excessive amount of fat in the body. This term is non-specific and is being replaced by a figure calculated from height and weight measurements, known as the **body mass index**.

Oncologist   A physician specialising in the treatment of tumours, particularly cancer.

Oncology   The study and management of new growths; the study of cancer.

Palliative therapy   Treatment used to alleviate symptoms but which cannot cure the condition which causes them.

Papilloma   A benign, stalked tumour of the epithelium.

Partial thickness skin graft   *See* Split-thickness skin graft.

Plastic surgeon   A surgeon specialising in the repair or reconstruction of acquired or congenital defects, with particular emphasis on restoring both function and appearance.

Post-operative   Following an operation.

Pre-clerking admission procedure   A procedure used in some hospitals whereby patients attend an appointment a few days before an operation for any necessary pre-operative tests, such as blood tests and ECGs, the results of which are thus available when the patient is admitted for surgery.

Predisposing risk factor   An environmental factor or characteristic present in an individual which increases his or her chances of developing a particular disease or condition.

Pre-malignant   Having malignant potential. A pre-malignant lesion may develop into a cancer, but does not necessarily do so.

Pre-medication ('Pre-med.')   A drug which is given before another drug, for example one given an hour or two before an operation to relax the patient before anaesthesia is started.

Pre-operative   Before an operation.

Primary tumour   The first (and sometimes only) or most important tumour to develop.

Prognosis   An opinion about the probable course and final outcome of a disease which is made when all the known facts are considered.

Pulmonary embolism   A blood clot or air bubble which blocks the blood vessels in the lung.

Pyrexia   A fever.

Radical treatment   Aggressive treatment aimed at curing a serious illness.

Radiographer   A technician qualified to make X-ray examinations.

Radiologist   A doctor trained in the use of X-radiation for diagnostic purposes.

Radiotherapist   A doctor specialising in the use of radiation as treatment, for example for cancer.

Radiotherapy   Treatment with radiation.

Reconstructive surgery   Surgery to repair and rebuild a damaged body part.

Recovery room   A ward near the operating theatre to which patients are taken after surgery so that they can be closely watched while they recover from a general anaesthetic.

Recurrence   The reappearance of symptoms or signs of a disease after a period of apparent recovery.

Regional chemotherapy   *See* Isolated limb perfusion.

Regional metastasis   Spread of malignant cells to nearby sites, usually the nearest lymph nodes.

Regression   The disappearance or reduction of the symptoms and signs of a disease.

Risk factor   Anything which increases the chances of developing a particular disease or condition. Risk factors include attributes which are already present, such as genes inherited from members of one's family, or can be acquired, such as smoking.

Rodent ulcer   A colloquial name for a basal cell carcinoma, so called because it sometimes has a rather ragged, 'chewed' appearance.

Sarcoma   A relatively rare cancer of the connective tissue.

Sebaceous gland   A gland within the dermis of the skin which secretes an oily substance (sebum) which lubricates the hair and skin surface.

Seborrhoeic keratosis/Basal cell papilloma/Senile wart/Seborrhoeic wart   A benign, wart-like skin lesion which is usually pigmented and often develops on a sun-exposed part of the body.

Secondary tumour   A tumour at a site distant from that of the original (primary) tumour; a metastasis.

Senile lentigo/Solar lentigo   A very large, benign freckle.

Senile wart   *See* Seborrhoeic keratosis.

Seroma   A collection of clear fluid, such as lymph, which may develop following an operation. If persistent, the fluid can be drawn off with a needle.

Side-effect An effect other than that desired which results from the use of a drug or other form of treatment.

Sign Something a doctor looks for as an indication of disease, such as a lesion or swelling.

Skin flap A layer of skin surgically separated from its underlying structures and repositioned to cover another adjacent site where the skin has been lost following injury or surgery.

Skin graft A piece of skin taken from one site on the body to replace that which has been lost because of injury or surgery at another site.

Solar keratosis *See* Actinic keratosis.

Solar lentigo *See* Senile lentigo.

Spinal anaesthetic An anaesthetic which is injected between the vertebrae of the spine into the space around the nerves in the back. It causes numbness in the legs and groin which lasts for three to five hours.

Split-thickness skin graft/Partial-thickness skin graft A graft of skin comprising epidermis and some dermis. It can be thin, intermediate or thick, depending on the depth of dermis included.

Squamous cell A flattened, scale-like cell within the epidermis of the skin.

Staging Classification of the development of a disease or condition. The stage at which a cancer is first detected may have a bearing on the likely outcome of its treatment.

Step-down ward A ward to which day-case patients may be taken in some hospitals to recover before going home after surgery.

Subcutaneous Under the skin.

Subcuticular Under the upper layer of the skin.

Sunblock A substance which is often opaque and which, when put on the skin, forms a film providing a physical or chemical barrier to ultraviolet radiation, preventing the skin from burning and tanning. Sun blocks are often white or coloured creams.

Sun protection factor (SPF)   A measure of the ability of a sunscreen preparation to reduce the exposure of the skin to ultraviolet radiation. The higher the SPF value, the greater the protection given to the skin and the longer it can be exposed to the sun before it burns.

Sunscreen preparation   A cream or lotion which is invisible on the skin, and which absorbs ultraviolet radiation before it reaches the epidermis, increasing the amount of time the skin can be exposed to the sun without burning.

Suntan preparation   A cream or lotion containing a chemical which reacts with chemicals in the skin to produce a colour resembling a tan. Unless the preparation has an SPF value, it will not protect the skin from sunburn.

Sun wart   *See* Actinic keratosis.

Suture   A surgical stitch or row of stitches.

Sweat gland   A gland within the dermis of the skin which secretes a watery fluid containing waste products from the body. The fluid passes through a duct onto the surface of the skin, from where it evaporates.

Symptom   Something experienced by a patient which indicates a disturbance of normal body function, for example pain or nausea.

Systemic injection   Injection of a substance which circulates around the body.

Telangiectasia   A condition involving multiple dilated blood vessels which may form a swelling.

Thrombo-embolic deterrent stockings (TEDS)   *See* Anti-embolism stockings.

Thrombosis   The coagulation of blood within a vein or artery which produces a blood clot.

Thrombus   A blood clot which forms in, and remains in, a blood vessel or the heart.

Tumour   A swelling; an abnormal growth of cells which can be benign or malignant. A *benign* tumour remains localised and does not spread to other parts of the body. It has no harmful effect except possibly to compress adjacent organs as it enlarges. A *malignant tumour* (a cancer) will invade the surrounding tissues, interfering with their normal functioning; cells from it may also spread to other parts of the body, giving rise to secondary tumours.

Tumour necrosis factor (TNF)   One of a group of **cytokines**, proteins which are produced by the body to control cell growth and death.

Ulcer   A lesion of the skin in which the surface layers have been destroyed, exposing the deeper tissues.

Ultraviolet radiation   Rays from the sun which are beyond the visible spectrum of light and are necessary for normal growth, but which in excess can cause damage to the skin.

Xeroderma pigmentosa   A rare genetic condition which involves extreme sensitivity of the skin to the sun. It becomes manifest in infancy or childhood as a blistering of exposed areas of the skin, and progresses to pigmentation and ulceration, and eventually to the development of skin cancer.

X-ray   A type of electromagnetic radiation of short wavelength which is able to pass through opaque bodies. It can be used in diagnosis, by allowing the visualisation of internal structures and organs of the body, or in higher doses as therapy to destroy malignant cells.

How to complain

If you are unhappy about anything that has occurred – or, indeed, that has not occurred – during your stay in hospital, there are several possible paths to follow if you want to make a complaint. However, the vast majority of complaints result from a failure of communication and many could be dealt with immediately if they are raised with the staff directly concerned. It is always best in the first instance to try to explain as clearly and unemotionally as possible what it is that you feel has gone wrong. If you do not feel able to discuss things directly, you may prefer to present your case in a letter. However angry or irritated you may feel, you are likely to find that a complaint made aggressively, however justified this may seem, is unlikely to achieve much.

If you are unable to achieve a satisfactory resolution of your problem in this way, you should give careful thought to what is involved before you set the complaints machinery in motion. Once a formal complaint has been made against a doctor and the complaints procedure has begun, there is little chance of stopping it.

The vast majority of doctors – family doctors and those who work in hospitals – are dedicated, conscientious and hard working. They really do have their patients' best interests at heart, and many work very long hours each week, night and day. A complaint against a doctor is usually a devastating blow, which can cause considerable stress. Of course, if something has gone wrong during your medical treatment, you may also have suffered stress and unhappiness, but before you make an official complaint, do consider whether your doctor's actions have really warranted what many would see as a 'kick in the teeth'.

The following sections explain briefly how to make an official complaint in the UK. The process will vary from country to country, but leaflets and other information giving details of all the appropriate councils and complaints procedures and how they work can be obtained from your hospital or local health authority. If you have any problems with the offices mentioned below, information about what to do and who to go to for help is available from Citizens' Advice Bureaus and Community Health Councils.

HOSPITAL STAFF

If your complaint concerns something that has happened during your stay in hospital, and for some reason you are unable to approach the person directly concerned, you can talk to the ward sister or charge nurse, the hospital doctor on your ward, your consultant or the senior manager for the department or ward. Many complaints can be dealt with directly by one of these people, but if this is not possible, they will be able to refer you to the appropriate person.

THE GENERAL MANAGER

If you are intimidated by the thought of speaking to one of the people mentioned above, you can write to the hospital's General Manager, sometimes called the Director of Operations or Chief Executive. The General Manager has responsibility for the way the hospital is run.

The Government's Patients' Charter states that anyone making a complaint about an NHS service must receive a 'full and prompt written reply from the Chief Executive or General Manager'. You should therefore receive an immediate response to your letter, and your complaint should be fully investigated by a senior manager.

The hospital switchboard, or any medical or clerical staff at the hospital, should be able to give you the General Manager's name and office address. If you would prefer to do so, you can make an appointment to speak to him or her, rather than writing a letter.

Depending on the seriousness of your complaint, you should receive either a full report of the investigation into it, or regular letters telling you what is happening until such a report can be made.

Do make sure you keep copies of all letters you write and receive concerning your complaint.

DISTRICT HEALTH AUTHORITY

If the treatment you require is not available in your area, or the waiting list is very long, you can contact your local District Health Authority. It is able to deal with complaints concerning the provision of services, rather than with those resulting from something going wrong with your treatment. The District Health Authority can sometimes arrange for you to have treatment elsewhere where waiting lists are shorter, if this is what you want.

Your NHS authority should produce a leaflet to explain how it deals with complaints. This will be available at your hospital or clinic. If you have any difficulty finding out who to contact, write to the General Manager of the hospital. Someone at the hospital will be able to tell you which health authority covers the area in which you live.

COMMUNITY HEALTH COUNCIL

Independent advice and assistance can be obtained from your local Community Health Council. Someone from the

Community Health Council will be able to explain the complaints procedures to you, help you to write letters to the hospital, and also come with you to any meetings arranged between hospital representatives and yourself. Again, the address of the Community Health Council for your area can be obtained from a hospital or local telephone directory.

REGIONAL MEDICAL OFFICER

If your complaint concerns the standard of *clinical* treatment you received in hospital, and the paths you have already taken have not led to a satisfactory conclusion, you can take it to the Regional Medical Officer for your area.

FAMILY HEALTH SERVICES AUTHORITY

Family doctors are now encouraged to have their own 'in-house' complaints services, but if you have a complaint about your family doctor which you have been unable to sort out by this means, it can be reported to the Family Health Services Authority. Such complaints should be made within 13 weeks of the incident occurring. Again, your local Community Health Council will be able to give you advice, help you make your complaint, and help you to write letters etc.

HEALTH SERVICE COMMISSIONER

If all else has failed, you can take your complaint to the Health Service Commissioner, who deals with complaints made by individuals against the NHS. The commissioner is independent of both the NHS and the Government, being responsible to Parliament.

The Health Service Commissioner is able to deal with complaints concerning the failure of an NHS authority to provide the service it should – a failure which has caused you actual hardship or injustice. However, you must have taken your complaint up with your Local Health Authority first. If you have not received a satisfactory response within a reasonable time, you must enclose copies of *all* the relevant letters and documents as well as giving details of the incident itself when writing to the Health Service Commissioner. The Health Commissioner is not able to investigate complaints about clinical treatment.

You must contact the Health Service Commissioner within *one year* of the incident occurring, unless there is some valid reason why you have been unable to do so.

There is a separate Health Service Commissioner for each country within the United Kingdom.

Health Service Commissioner for England
Church House
Great Smith Street
London SW1P 3BW
Telephone: 0171 276 2035

Health Service Commissioner for Scotland
Second Floor
11 Melville Crescent
Edinburgh EH3 7LU
Telephone: 0131 225 7465

Health Service Commissioner for Wales
4th Floor Pearl Assurance House
Greyfriars Road
Cardiff CF1 3AG
Telephone: 01222 394621

Office of the Northern Ireland Commissioner for Complaints
33 Wellington Place
Belfast BT1 6HN
Telephone: 01232 233821

TAKING LEGAL ACTION

The legal path is likely to be an expensive one, and should be a last resort rather than a starting point.

In theory, everyone has a right to take legal action. However, unless you have very little money and are entitled to Legal Aid, or a great deal of money, you are unlikely to be able to afford this costly process. The outcome of legal action can never be assured, and the possible cost if you lose your case should be borne in mind.

If you do think you have grounds for compensation for injury caused to you as a result of negligence, advice can be sought from:

The Association for the Victims of Medical Accidents (AVMA)
1 London Road
Forest Hill
London SE23 3TP
Telephone: 0181 291 2793.

Someone from the AVMA will be able to give you free and confidential legal advice about whether or not you have a case worth pursuing. They will also be able to recommend solicitors with training in medical law who may be prepared to represent you.

SUMMARY

Do tell nursing or other medical staff if you are not happy about *any* aspect of your care in hospital. They may be able to deal with your complaint immediately. But do remember, if your complaint is about a serious matter, or if you are not satisfied with the response you receive, you are entitled to pursue it through all the levels that exist to deal with such problems.

Useful addresses

The organisations listed here provide a range of services, including advice and information about skin cancer and about the help available to sufferers and their families.

GREAT BRITAIN

The Skin Cancer Research Fund
Department of Plastic Surgery
Frenchay Hospital
Frenchay
Bristol BS16 1LE
Telephone: 0117 9701212, Extension 3130

Skin Care Campaign
163 Eversholt Street
London NW1 1BU
Telephone: 0171 388 5655

Outlook
Disfigurement Support Unit
Ward 6
Frenchay Hospital
Bristol BS16 1LE
Telephone: 0117 9701212, Extension 2306

British Red Cross
9 Grosvenor Crescent
London SW1X 7EJ
Telephone: 0171 2355454

Cancer Research Campaign
6–10 Cambridge Terrace
Regent's Park
London NW1 4JL
Telephone: 0171 224 1333

The British Association of Cancer-United Patients (BACUP)
3 Bath Place
Rivington Street
London EC2A 3JR
Phone 0171 613 2121
Freephone counselling service for patients: 0800 181199

Cancerlink
17 Britannia Street
London WC1X 9JN
Telephone: 0171 833 2451

9 Castle Terrace
Edinburgh EH1 2DP
Telephone: 0131 228 557

Cancer Aftercare and Rehabilitation Society (CARE)
21 Zetland Road
Redland
Bristol BS6 7AH
Telephone: 0117 9427419

Cancer Relief Macmillan Fund
Anchor House
15/19 Britten Street
London SW3 3TZ
Telephone: 0171 351 7811

Carers' National Association
29 Chilworth Mews
London W2 3RG
Telephone: 0171 724 7776

Hospice Information Service
St Christopher's Hospice
51–59 Lawrie Park Road
Sydenham
London SE26 6DZ
Telephone: 0181 778 9252

Institute for Complementary Medicine
PO Box 194
London SE16 1Q2

Irish Cancer Society
Information Officer
5 Northumberland Road
Dublin 4
Telephone: 1 681855
Helpline: 1 681233

The Ulster Cancer Foundation
40–42 Eglantine Avenue
Belfast BT9 6DX
Telephone: 01232 663281/2/3
Helpline: 01232 663449

Tak Tent Cancer Support Organisation
G Block
Western Infirmary
Glasgow G11 6NT
Telephone: 0141 334 6699 or 0141 357 4519

Tenovus Cancer Information Centre
142 Whitchurch Road
Cardiff CF4 3NA
Telephone: 01222 619846
Helpline: 01222 691998

AUSTRALIA

Skin Cancer Foundation
277 Bourke Street
Darlinghurst
New South Wales 2010
Telephone: 02 360 4480

Australian Cancer Society
Angus & Coote Building
500 George Street
Sydney
New South Wales 2000
Telephone: 02 267 1944

Anti-Cancer Council of Victoria
1 Rathdowne Street
Carlton
South Victoria 3053
Telephone: 03 662 3300

Anti-Cancer Foundation of the Universities of South Australia
24 Brougham Place
North Adelaide
South Australia 5006
Telephone: 08 267 5222

Cancer Foundation of Western Australia Inc.
42 Ord Street
West Perth
Western Australia 6005
Telephone: 09 321 6224

Northern Territory Anti-Cancer Foundation
Shop 24
Casuarina Plaza
Casuarina
Northern Territory 0810
Telephone: 08 927 4888

Queensland Cancer Fund
553 Gregory Terrace
Fortitude Valley
Queensland 4006
Telephone: 07 257 1155

Tasmanian Cancer Committee
43 Collins Street
Hobart
Tasmania 7000
Telephone: 002 30 0895

NEW ZEALAND

Cancer Society of New Zealand Inc.
Molesworthy House
101–105 Molesworthy Street
P.O. Box 12145
Wellington
New Zealand
Telephone: 4 473 6409

CANADA

The **Canadian Cancer Society** is a national organization with the following offices throughout the country.

Chimo Building, 2nd Floor
P.O. Box 8921
Freshwater & Crosbie Road
St John's
Newfoundland A1B 3R9
Telephone: 709 753 6520

1 Rochford Street, Suite #1
Charlottetown
Prince Edward Island C1A 3T1
Telephone: 902 566 4007
5826 South Street, Suite 1
Halifax
Nova Scotia B3H 1S6
Telephone: 902 423 6183

133 Prince William Street
P.O. Box 2089
Saint John
New Brunswick E2L 3T6
Telephone: 506 634 6272

Maison de la societe canadienne du cancer
5151 Boul. l'Assumption
Montreal
Quebec H1T 4A9
Telephone: 514 255 5151

1639 Yonge Street
Toronto
Ontario M4T 2W6
Telephone: 416 488 5400

193 Sherbrook Street
Winnipeg
Manitoba R3C 2B7
Telephone: 204 774 7483

2445 13th Avenue, Suite 201
Regina
Saskatchewan S4P 0W1
Telephone: 306 757 4260
#200, 2424 4th Street S.W.
Calgary
Alberta T2S 2T4
Telephone: 403 228 4487

565 West Tenth Avenue
Vancouver
British Columbia V5Z 4J4
Telephone: 604 872 4400

NORTH AMERICA

There are too many organizations throughout the USA to list
them all here. The following are just a few examples. Your local
State Department of Health should be able to supply further
addresses of centers in your area.

Skin Cancer Foundation
245 Fifth Avenue
New York
New York 10016
Telephone: 212 725 5176

Melanoma Foundation
750 Menlo Avenue
Suite 250
Menlo Park
California 94025

American Cancer Society
1599 Clifton Road NE
Atlanta
Georgia 30329
Telephone: 404 320 3333

Cancer Care
1180 Avenue of the Americas
New York
New York 10036
Telephone: 212 221 3300

Cancer Information Service
Office of Cancer Communication
NCI/NIH, Buildin 31, 10A07
9000 Rockville Pike
Bethesda
Maryland 20892

Cancer Control Society
2043 N. Berendo Street
Los Angeles
California 90027
Telephone: 213 663 7801

International Health Council
P.O. Box 151
Fairbanks
Alaska 99707

R.A. Bloch Cancer Foundation
4410 Main
Kansas City
Missouri 64111
Telephone: 816 932 8453

Index

linear accelerator 83, 84
local anaesthesia 57-8
lymphoedema 94
lymph nodes 1
 excision of 68-9
  swelling after 81
 spread of cancer to 1,
  89
lymphoma 8

Macmillan nurses 98
malignant melanoma 7,
 11-15
 biopsy of 33
 chemotherapy for 92-4
 immunotherapy for
  94-5
 invasion of 13-14
 metastasis of 13, 88-9
 pregnancy and 35
 radiotherapy for 82
 treatment of 14-15,
  36-8
melanin 3, 25
melanocytes 3
melanoma, see malignant
 melanoma
metastasis 1-2, 88-9
microvascular flaps 68
Mohs chemotherapy 37
moles (see also naevi) 5, 30

naevi 4-5, 6
nerve block 58
neuroma 81
neuropathy 93
nil by mouth 54, 60
numbness, see paraesthesia

obesity, and surgery 54-5
oncologist 32, 90
operations, see surgery

painkillers 62, 74-5
pain
 post-operative 79, 80
 relief of 62
palliation 96-9
paraesthesia 81
physiotherapy 75
pin cushion effect 81
plastic surgeon 32, 35
pregnancy, and malignant
 melanoma 35

pre-medication 53, 59,
 60
private care 100-107
private health insurance
 101-102
pulmonary embolism 50,
 79
pyrexia, post-operative 80

radiographer 82, 85
radiologist 82
radiotherapist 82
radiotherapy 35, 38, 82-7
 as adjuvant 90
 side-effects of 87
recovery room 61
recurrent disease 88
regional chemotherapy 93
risk factors for skin cancer
 15-19, 22
rodent ulcer (see also basal
 cell carcinoma) 8

sarcoma 8
scabs 85
scars
 after excision 32
 after radiotherapy 87
 camouflage of 87
 complications of 81
sclerosing angioma 6
seborrhoeic keratosis 5
seborrhoeic wart 5
self-examination 28-9
senile lentigo 5
senile wart 5
seroma 80
signs
 of deep vein thrombosis
  79
 of pulmonary embolism
  79
 of skin cancer 30-31
skin 2-4
skin care
 after radiotherapy 86-7
 after surgery 72-3
skin flaps 68, 69
 post-operative care of
  71-6
skin grafts 65-7, 72
 care of donor site 73
 care of post-operatively
  71-2, 76

partial thickness 67
 full thickness 67
 split-thickness 67
smoking, and surgery 54
solar keratosis 6
solar lentigo 5
spinal anaesthetic 57-8
squamous cell carcinoma
 10-11
 chemotherapy for 91
 radiotherapy for 82-7
 treatment of 36, 37-8
step-down ward 61
stitches 65
 removal of 75-6
sun (see also ultraviolet
 radiation)
 protecting skin from
  23-7
 role of in skin cancer
  15-17
sunbeds 28
sunblocks 25
sunburn 23-7
sunglasses 27
sunscreen preparations
 25-7
sunscreen protection
 factors (SPFs) 26
suntan preparations
 26-7
sun wart 6
surgery 36, 63-9
sutures, see stitches

telangiectasia 87
tests, pre-operative 41,
 49
thrombo-embolic deterrent
 stockings (TEDS) 50-51,
 78-9
thrombosis 50, 78-9
thrombus, see blood clots

ultraviolet radiation
 15-17, 24, 25, 27
 and sunbeds 28

wounds 71-3
 infection of 80

X-rays (see also radiotherapy)
 83